The Pathophysiology and Treatment

of

DROWNING AND NEAR-DROWNING

The Pathophysiology and Treatment

of

DROWNING AND NEAR-DROWNING

By

JEROME H. MODELL, M.D.

Professor and Chairman
Department of Anesthesiology
University of Florida College of Medicine
Gainesville, Florida

With a Foreword by

Frank Moya, M.D.

Professor and Chairman
Department of Anesthesiology
Associate Dean
University of Miami School of Medicine
Miami, Florida

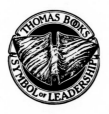

CHARLES C THOMAS • PUBLISHER
Springfield • Illinois • U.S.A.

Published and Distributed Throughout the World by

CHARLES C THOMAS • PUBLISHER

BANNERSTONE HOUSE

301-327 East Lawrence Avenue, Springfield, Illinois, U.S.A.

NATCHEZ PLANTATION HOUSE

735 North Atlantic Boulevard, Fort Lauderdale, Florida, U.S.A.

With **THOMAS BOOKS** *careful attention is given to all details of manufacturing and design. It is the Publisher's desire to present books that are satisfactory as to their physical qualities and artistic possibilities and appropriate for their particular use.* **THOMAS BOOKS** *will be true to those laws of quality that assure a good name and good will.*

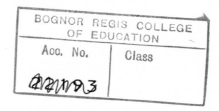
Printed in the United States of America

A-2

To

MISS KAY DIDICH

whose gallant fight for life fell short, but whose clinical course stimulated the author and his colleagues to perform many of the studies summarized in this text

CONTRIBUTORS

THE AUTHOR WISHES TO THANK Joseph H. Davis, M.D., Medical Examiner of Dade County, Professor of Legal Medicine, University of Miami School of Medicine, Miami, Florida, for contributing Chapters XI and XII; and H. Dennison Williams, M.D., of Clermont, Florida, for collaborating on Chapter I.

FOREWORD

Drowning accounts for over 7,000 deaths each year in the United States alone. Indeed, drowning now ranks as one of the three leading causes of accidental death. Hopefully, a better understanding of the pathophysiological principles involved and better education of those who must care for near-drowning victims will lead to a reduction in these grim statistics.

Interestingly enough, it was one such case that led ultimately to the writing of this book. The very first experience Dr. Modell had with a drowning victim was a Japanese naval officer who was found unconscious at the bottom of a swimming pool. The apparent discrepancy between the officer's blood picture and information available in the literature at the time stimulated his curiosity and led eventually to the initial experiments on drowning and near-drowning.

Dr. Modell has drawn on his considerable experience in the laboratory and intensive care unit to prepare a book which crosses many disciplinary lines. This excellent text, the only volume currently available dealing with the complete problem of drowning and near-drowning, should be of great interest to physicians, rescue workers, paramedical personnel, and physiologists as well. It is an important contribution to the scientific literature and should stand as a classic reference for years to come.

FRANK MOYA, M. D.

PREFACE

In 1962, I suddenly was faced with having to treat a physician who near-drowned in fresh water. This patient was severely ill and had aspirated a significant quantity of water. However, analysis of his blood did not reveal the marked shifts in serum electrolyte concentrations, hemoglobin, or hematocrit that would have been predicted from animal studies that were reported during the preceding twenty-five years. The following year, a retrospective report by Fuller of electrolyte findings in human near-drowning victims also failed to demonstrate a significant deviation from normal. This led us to question whether the response of animals to drowning and near-drowning might be different from that of humans, or whether the experimental conditions in prior animal studies were comparable to the conditions experienced by humans.

Later that year, I joined the faculty at the University of Miami School of Medicine, which enabled me and my colleagues in the Department of Anesthesiology to pursue studies aimed at answering these questions. The studies performed in that laboratory, as well as those subsequently performed at the University of Florida, correlate very well with observations during the treatment of human near-drowning victims. There is not a discrepancy between animals and humans. Rather, they must be studied under comparable conditions.

This text has been written in an attempt to bring together most of what is known in the literature regarding the pathophysiology and treatment of this disease. It is hoped that this text will serve its purpose of tying together animal experiments with human observations, in order to produce a better understanding of the disease and a logical method of therapy based upon sound physiologic principles.

ACKNOWLEDGMENTS

THE ORIGINAL STUDIES in this field conducted by the author and his colleagues were made possible through grants from the United Health Foundation of Dade County, National Science Foundation NSF/GU-0728 Sub IX, and U. S. Public Health Service NIH-GM12154, NIH-1K3-GM33840, and NIH-GM17246.

There are many people whose efforts and suggestions led to the preparation of this work. To Doctor Frank Moya, Professor and Chairman of the Department of Anesthesiology at the University of Miami School of Medicine, I express my grateful appreciation. His support, encouragement, and guidance not only made these studies possible but also were the primary factors in shaping this author's career in academic medicine.

I also wish to express my sincere gratitude to Mrs. Carol-Joan Sullivan, who first suggested writing this book, and who provided secretarial support for preparing multiple drafts; to Mr. Bruce C. Ruiz, Mrs. Earlene J. Kuck, and Miss April V. Showers, who assisted in gathering much of the data incorporated within the text; to Doctor Thorkild W. Andersen and Miss Pamela M. Warwick, whose editorial suggestions were most helpful in preparing the manuscript; and finally, to my wife Marilyn for her patience, understanding, and inspiration.

J.H.M.

CONTENTS

The Pathophysiology and Treatment

of

DROWNING AND NEAR-DROWNING

Chapter 1

STATISTICS AND PUBLIC HEALTH CONSIDERATIONS

H. DENNISON WILLIAMS AND JEROME H. MODELL

FROM 1947 to 1967 over 110,000 persons died of drowning in the United States[1] (Table I). Drowning thus ranked as one of the three leading causes of accidental death.[2-4] In Great Britain, the number of deaths from drowning was approximately 1,100 per annum, while Australia and Norway reported 500 each.[2,5-7] Impressive as these figures are, they do not reflect the vast numbers of

TABLE I

DEATHS AND DEATH RATES FROM DROWNING
UNITED STATES, 1947-1967

Year	Numbers	Rates
1967	5,724	2.9
1966	5,687	2.9
1965	5,485	2.8
1964	5,433	2.8
1963	5,103	2.7
1962	5,161	2.8
1961	5,208	2.8
1960	5,232	2.9
1959	5,046	2.9
1958	5,065	2.9
1957	5,209	3.1
1956	4,902	2.9
1955	5,046	3.1
1954	5,049	3.1
1953	5,352	3.4
1952	5,346	3.4
1951	5,055	3.3
1950	4,785	3.2
1949	5,330	3.6
1948	5,299	3.6
1947	5,737	4.0
	Total 110,254	

Courtesty of the Department of Health, Education, and Welfare Public Health Service, National Center for Health Statistics, Washington, D. C., 20201.

3

TABLE II

NUMBER OF DROWNINGS BY SITE, AGE GROUP AND PER CENT MALE IN COLORADO, FLORIDA, ILLINOIS, NEW YORK, AND NORTH CAROLINA: JULY 1, 1965-JUNE 30, 1966

	All ages		0-4		5-9		10-19		20-29		30-39		40-49		50-64		65+		NR**	
Site	Total	% Male	Total	% Male	Total	% Male	Total	% Male	Total	% Male	Total	% Male	Total	% Male	Total	% Male	Total	% Male	Total	% Male
Total	1,201	85	126	76	100	82	292	88	144	88	90	87	122	87	154	85	98	81	75	84
River	298	87	9	56	15	80	52	87	40	93	41	88	43	86	51	92	29	76	18	94
Quarry	31	97	2	100	2	100	16	94	3	100	1	100	4	100	....	0	....	0	3	100
Lake	275	89	15	93	19	84	84	92	49	86	20	85	26	96	34	88	15	93	13	77
Pond	130	89	11	82	18	89	50	94	11	100	5	80	8	88	12	75	5	100	10	70
Public swimming pool	30	83	3	33	4	100	14	79	2	100	....	0	1	100	1	100	4	100	1	100
Private fenced pool	24	83	13	85	2	100	5	60	....	0	1	100	....	0	1	100	1	100	1	100
Private unfenced pool	17	59	8	63	1	100	3	33	....	0	....	0	....	0	2	100	2	50	1	0
Bathtub	62	58	27	70	1	100	2	50	3	33	3	67	6	17	7	43	8	50	5	80
Ocean	85	87	....	0	7	86	16	94	13	85	6	83	8	88	12	92	14	79	9	89
Other	210	84	31	77	28	75	43	84	18	89	11	91	21	95	28	82	18	89	12	83
Gulf*	4	75	....	0	....	0	2	100	2	50	....	0	....	0	....	0	....	0	....	0
Canal*	35	80	7	86	3	33	5	100	3	100	2	100	5	80	6	67	2	50	2	100

Modified with permission from *AJPH*, 58:12, 1968, published by the American Public Health Association.

*Category used for Florida incidents only.

**NR = not reported.

persons who "near-drowned" and recovered. With the current explosive growth of the aquatic industry and water sports, an increased incidence of drowning is predicted for the future.[8-11]

The highest incidence of death from drowning occurs in persons from ten to nineteen years of age[2,8,9,11] (Table II). However, neither the very young nor the elderly are spared from drowning, e.g. approximately 400 children under two years old drown annually.[4,12] Over half of the victims of drowning in swimming pools in the United States are children under ten.[13] Similar statistics are reported from the United Kingdom where 42 percent of accidental drownings occurred in children under sixteen.[7] Males accounted for 85 percent of the deaths from drowning reported by Press, Walker, and Crawford.[11]

Immediately preceding death from drowning, victims were noted to be swimming, playing, power boating, and fishing, in that order. Although proficiency in swimming unquestionably is desirable, reports show that as many as 35 percent of drowning victims could swim.[8,11] The factors which offset a person's ability to swim were over-confidence, attempts to swim long distances, and the desire to bolster one's ego by showing-off.[11] This may explain the considerably higher incidence of drowning in males as they may have been trying to advertise their masculinity. Unattended children playing near the edges of rivers, canals, or pools comprised the majority of victims in the second category. Fatalities while boating and fishing were usually related to a disregard of safety rules, especially the failure to use life preservers. Of 166 victims of drowning while boating, only five persons wore a life preserver and stayed with the boat. Three of these used their life preserver improperly.[11]

The number of people taking up the sports of skin diving and scuba diving is increasing rapidly; by now 8 million people skin dive and another million use scuba diving equipment in the United States. Therefore, it is not surprising that these sports are becoming a significant contributing factor to deaths from drowning. Most accidents and deaths from skin diving or scuba diving have been attributed to inexperience or lack of adequate training.[10]

Although most of the state of Florida is surrounded by ocean beaches, the greatest incidence of drowning occurs not at the beaches but in rivers and canals. Mishaps in lakes rank second and drowning at beaches only third. The order is similar in other states,[11] as well as in Great Britain where canals and rivers claim 77 percent of drowning victims.[7] Swimming pools are the most frequent site of infant drownings. Lack of adequate enclosures and improper supervision of pools have been linked with more than half of all pool drownings.[13] Most elderly people who succumb from drowning die in the bathtub,[8,13] and it is not always possible to determine whether drowning or cardiovascular collapse is the primary cause of death.[11] As might be expected, summer is the peak season for deaths from drowning, and they occur most frequently during the daylight hours on weekends.[5,10,11,13]

Thirty-six percent of 2,577 victims of drowning or near-drowning, reported in five surveys, received artificial ventilation.[6,7,10,11,13] In most cases, the length of time between the onset of submersion and the start of artificial ventilation was not reported. In the more recent reports, mouth-to-mouth ventilation and mechanically operated devices were employed most frequently, whereas external chest compression was used in the past.[6,7,11] The reason often stated for the failure to resuscitate drowning victims is that the person remained in the water too long prior to discovery. This may be true in many cases, but frequently, resuscitative efforts were not instituted immediately after recovery of the body, were not continued for a sufficient period of time, or were performed incorrectly.[6,10,11,13]

The fact that 157 deaths from drowning occurred in the United States over the 1969 Memorial Day weekend alone indicates that this is a serious problem and that there is a need for improvement in the prevention of these accidents and in the treatment of the victims. Apparently, little benefit has been achieved by warnings issued to the public such as "be careful while swimming or boating." Statistics indicate that children and young adults can benefit most from educational programs.[5] Irresponsible action could be decreased by impressing mothers with mortality figures for unattended infants.[14] Parents and guardians should be prompted to provide adequate supervision at swimming pools, beaches, and other areas, even though life guards may be present. All persons should become familiar with the dangers of panic and of attempting to rescue a drowning person.[3,4,8,11-13]

The above discussion emphasizes one fact: *the number of deaths due to drowning can be reduced.* However, in spite of intensified efforts at education, some people always will remain reckless and loss of life from aquatic accidents will continue. The ensuing chapters will summarize the most recent experimental and clinical information available in the hope that, with better understanding of the pathophysiology involved, the incidence of survival following drowning will increase and the morbidity after near-drowning will decrease.

REFERENCES

1. Zugzda, M. J.: Personal communication. July 25, 1969.
2. Boucher, C. A.: Drowning. *Monthly Bull Minist Health (London), 21:* 114-117, 1962.
3. Brown, R. L.: Prevention of water accidents. A half century reviewed. *Public Health Rep, 69:*575-580, 1954.
4. Baker, A. Z.: Drowning and swimming. *Practitioner, 172:*655-659, 1954.
5. Adams, A. I.: The descriptive epidemiology of drowning accidents. *Med J Aust, 2:*1257-1261, 1966.
6. Lind, B., and Stovner, J.: Mouth-to-mouth resuscitation in Norway. *JAMA, 185:*933-935, 1963.
7. Hale, E.: Analysis of fatal drowning accidents which occurred in 1961. *J Roy Nav Med Serv, 49:*233-236, 1963.
8. Press, E.; Walker, J., and Crawford, I.: Preliminary study of Illinois drownings. *Illinois Med J, 127:*577-581, 1965.
9. Arkansas Public Health at a Glance: Deaths from accidental drowning. *Arkansas Med Society, 58:*65-66, 1961.
10. Webster, D. P.: Skin and scuba diving fatalities in the United States. *Public Health Rep, 81:*703-711, 1966.
11. Press, E.; Walker, J., and Crawford, I.: An interstate drowning study. *Amer J Public Health, 58:*2275-2289, 1968.
12. Curran, J.: Accidental drownings of infants. *New York J Med, 40:*1131, 1940.
13. Webster, D. P.: Pool drownings and their prevention. *Public Health Rep, 82:*587-600, 1967.
14. Spitz, W. U., and Blanke, R. V.: Mechanism of death in fresh-water drowning. I. An experimental approach to the problem. *Arch Path (Chicago), 71:*661-668, 1961.

Chapter II

DEFINITIONS AND DESCRIPTIONS

DEFINITIONS

THERE APPEARS TO BE some confusion and apparent inconsistency between data obtained during experimental drowning of animals and observations in humans. Much of this may be attributed to the use of the term *to drown* as being all inclusive. Webster's Dictionary defines "drown" as "to suffocate by submersion, especially in water."[1] It has been estimated that approximately 10 percent of the victims of drowning do not actually aspirate water. They die from acute asphyxia, while submerged, due to reflex laryngospasm.[2,3] Since the pathophysiological changes in these patients are considerably different from those in patients who have aspirated fluid, at least two subdefinitions of "drown" are necessary. The phrase *drown without aspiration* is proposed for patients who have died from respiratory obstruction and asphyxia while submerged in a fluid medium. *Drown with aspiration* is a more appropriate phrase for those who actually aspirate fluid.[4] It will become apparent in the ensuing chapters that the definition *drown with aspiration* must be further subdivided according to the type and volume of fluid that is aspirated.

Since "drown" implies death, and we are concerned primarily with resuscitation and survival, further modification of the definition is necessary to include "near-drowning." Redding, Voigt, and Safar have shown in animal experiments simulating *near-drowning without aspiration* that, if effective mechanical ventilation is instituted promptly, irreversible changes can be prevented.[5] If water is aspirated, however, a more complicated picture is seen. The magnitude and nature of the changes after *near-drowning with aspiration* depend, primarily, upon the quantity and composition of fluid aspirated.[6-8] The manner in which the volume and type of fluid aspirated influences the pathophysiological changes seen after a near-drowning episode will be discussed in detail in ensuing chapters.

The Standard Nomenclature of Athletic Injuries lists "near-drowning" as "a critical aquatic predicament resolved by successful water rescue."[9] This definition implies that recovery is certain once the victim is removed from the water. However, this is not always the case. Some patients who have regained consciousness after near-drowning, subsequently have died.[10,11] Countless others probably have met a similar fate, but have gone unreported. Ultimate survival should not be a consideration in the initial classification of these patients. The group of patients who are rescued alive or who are resuscitated, only to die later of their immersion episode, might be properly classified *delayed death subsequent to near-drowning.*

To understand this complex group of diseases more clearly, the following definitions are offered:

Drown without aspiration: To die from respiratory obstruction and asphyxia while submerged in a fluid medium.

Drown with aspiration: To die from the combined effects of asphyxia and changes secondary to aspiration of fluid while submerged.

Near-drowning without aspiration: To survive, at least temporarily, following asphyxia due to submersion in a fluid medium.

Near-drowning with aspiration: To survive, at least temporarily, following aspiration of fluid while submerged.

Delayed death subsequent to near-drowning: To succumb subsequent to near-drowning after apparent successful rescue or resuscitation.

DESCRIPTION OF DROWNING EPISODE

There is no agreement upon the exact sequence of events during a drowning episode, nor upon how long an animal or human can stay submerged and still survive. Karpovich,[12] through his studies of rats, guinea pigs, and cats, has shown the sequence of events during drowning to be (1) an immediate struggle for freedom; sometimes a surprise inhalation; (2) suspension of movement; exhalation of a little air and frequent swallowing; (3) a violent struggle for freedom; (4) convulsions; exhalation of air and spasmodic inspiratory efforts; disappearance of reflexes; and (5) death.

A description of the reaction of dogs to total immersion is reasonably similar. Lougheed, Janes, and Hall[13] described a period of breath-holding and struggling for approximately one and one-half minutes, which was followed by swallowing large amounts of water, gasping with aspiration, spasmodic struggling resembling tetanic convulsions, and violent vomiting. Finally, there was a loss of all movement and, within five minutes, apparent death.

Understandably, controlled observations in humans are lacking. It is likely that Noble and Sharpe's[14] reconstruction of the events which occur is reasonably accurate for many victims. These authors report that the patient panics, struggles violently, and then makes automatic swimming movements. Apnea, or breath-holding, occurs and the victim then swallows large amounts of water. Vomiting and gasping ensues and water is aspirated. Blood-stained froth appears in the airways, the patient convulses, and finally, dies. This sequence of events is also compatible with the personal experiences described by Lowson[15] after he near-drowned in 1892.

Although it would seem that an accomplished swimmer is less likely to drown than the nonswimmer, in recent years a number of cases has been reported of drowning and near-drowning by skilled swimmers.[16-21]

Usually, these accidents are associated with underwater swimming after hyperventilation. The sequence of events is quite different from that seen in the panicked nonswimmer. These individuals are observed to voluntarily hyperventilate immediately prior to attempting to reach a goal in length of underwater swimming. Suddenly, they are observed motionless on the bottom of the pool.

Some authors have implied that if consciousness is not lost during a near-drowning episode, complete recovery can be expected.[22] Yet, severe respiratory insufficiency can develop in patients who have aspirated fluid but have not lost consciousness.[23] Likewise, the return of consciousness is not synonymous with recovery, as delayed deaths have occurred.[10,11] Others have suggested that submersion for up to five minutes may be uniformly fatal.[13] However, survival of patients who have been treated after total submersion for ten minutes,[24] 17 minutes,[25] and even 22 minutes[26] has been reported!

It should be apparent that no two drowning or near-drowning

victims are alike. Obviously their age and previous state of health are important. The circumstances surrounding the accidents also may be considerably different. The physiologic state of the victim when rescued will depend somewhat upon the duration of submersion, but this cannot solely be used to determine the ultimate chances of survival. Perhaps even more importantly, the pathophysiologic changes seen will depend upon the type and volume of water aspirated by the victim. All these factors must be taken into account in the description of an individual patient. Therefore, I feel it is necessary to expand and subdivide the traditional definition of "drown."

REFERENCES

1. *Webster's Seventh New Collegiate Dictionary.* Springfield, Merriam, 1969, p. 255.
2. Cot, C.: *Les Asphyxies Accidentelles* (submersion, electrocution, intoxication oxycarbonique). Etude clinique, therapeutique et preventive. Paris, Editions medicales N. Maloine, 1931.
3. Moritz, A. R.: Chemical methods for the determination of death by drowning. *Physiol Rev, 24*:70-88, 1944.
4. Modell, J. H.: The pathophysiology and treatment of drowning. *Acta Anaesth Scand Suppl, 29*:263-279, 1968.
5. Redding, J.; Voigt, G. C., and Safar, P.: Drowning treated with intermittent positive pressure breathing. *J Appl Physiol, 15*:849-854, 1960.
6. Modell, J. H., and Moya, F.: Effects of volume of aspirated fluid during chlorinated fresh water drowning. *Anesthesiology, 27*:662-672, 1966.
7. Modell, J. H.; Gaub, M.; Moya, F.; Vestal, B., and Swarz, H.: Physiologic effects of near drowning with chlorinated fresh water, distilled water and isotonic saline. *Anesthesiology, 27*:33-41, 1966.
8. Modell, J. H.; Moya, F.; Newby, E. J.; Ruiz, B. C., and Showers, A. V.: The effects of fluid volume in seawater drowning. *Ann Intern Med, 67*:68-80, 1967.
9. Rachun, A.: *Standard Nomenclature of Athletic Injuries.* Chicago, American Medical Association, 1966, p. 125.
10. Wong, F. M., and Grace, W. J.: Sudden death after near-drowning. *JAMA, 186*:724-726, 1963.
11. Modell, J. H.; Davis, J. H.; Giammona, S. T.; Moya, F., and Mann, J. B.: Blood gas and electrolyte changes in human near-drowning victims. *JAMA, 203*:337-343, 1968.
12. Karpovich, P. V.: Water in the lungs of drowned animals. *Arch Path (Chicago), 15*:828-833, 1933.
13. Lougheed, D. W.; Janes, J. M., and Hall, G. E.: Physiological studies in experimental asphyxia and drowning. *Canad Med Ass J, 40*:423-428,

1939.

14. Noble, C. S., and Sharpe, N.: Drowning; its mechanism and treatment. *Canad Med Ass J, 89*:402-405, 1963.

15. Lowson, J. A.: Sensations in drowning. *Edinburgh Med J, 13*:41-45, 1903.

16. Munroe, W. D.: Hemoglobinuria from near-drowning. *J Pediat, 64*:57-62, 1964.

17. Craig, A. B., Jr.: Underwater swimming and loss of consciousness. *JAMA, 176*:255-258, 1961.

18. Dumitru, A. P., and Hamilton, F. G.: A mechanism of drowning. *Anesth Analg (Cleveland), 42*:170-176, 1963.

19. Craig, A. B., Jr.: Causes of loss of consciousness during underwater swimming. *J Appl Physiol, 16*:583-586, 1961.

20. Modell, J. H.: Resuscitation after aspiration of chlorinated fresh water. *JAMA, 185*:651-655, 1963.

21. Dumitru, A. P., and Hamilton, F. G.: Underwater blackout—a mechanism of drowning. *GP, 29*:123-125, 1964.

22. Cahill, J. M.: Drowning: the problem of nonfatal submersion and the unconscious patient. *Surg Clin N Amer, 48*:423-430, 1968.

23. Fainer, D. C.: Near drowning in sea water and fresh water. *Ann Intern Med, 59*:537-541, 1963.

24. Ohlsson, K., and Beckman, M.: Drowning—reflections based on two cases. *Acta Chir Scand, 128*:327-339, 1964.

25. King, R. B., and Webster, I. W.: A case of recovery from drowning and prolonged anoxia. *Med J Aust, 1*:919-920, 1964.

26. Kvittingen, T. D., and Naess, A.: Recovery from drowning in fresh water. *Brit Med J, 5341*:1315-1317, May, 1963.

Chapter III

BLOOD GAS AND ACID-BASE CHANGES

THE SINGLE MOST IMPORTANT CONSEQUENCE of near-drowning is *hypoxemia*. The degree and duration of hypoxemia depends upon the duration of submersion and whether or not the patient aspirates fluid. Initially, hypoxemia is accompanied by hypercarbia and acidosis. When fluid is aspirated, however, the hypoxemia persists, even after the pH and $PaCO_2$ have returned to normal.

DROWNING AND NEAR-DROWNING WITHOUT ASPIRATION

Initially, a mammal responds to total immersion in liquid by either closing his vocal cords (i.e. laryngospasm) or by holding his breath.[1-3] It has been estimated that approximately 10 percent of human drowning victims die during laryngospasm or breath-holding without actually aspirating fluid.[4] One approach to simulating laryngospasm experimentally is to occlude the endotracheal tube after an animal has been intubated. Table III illustrates the mean changes in arterial pH, Po_2, Pco_2 and base excess that occurred in a group of anesthetized dogs when airway obstruction was produced by this method. Progressive changes were seen in all

TABLE III

ARTERIAL BLOOD GAS AND pH VALUES PRIOR TO AND
FOLLOWING ACUTE TRACHEAL OBSTRUCTION*

Time (Minutes)	pHa	$PaCO_2$ torr	PaO_2 torr	Base Excess mEq/liter
0	7.45 ± .06	30 ± 5	92 ± 22	—1 ± 3
1	7.37 ± .06	36 ± 5	40 ± 6	—3 ± 2
3	7.32 ± .06	42 ± 5	10 ± 2	—4 ± 2
5	7.21 ± .06	48 ± 6	4 ± 1	—9 ± 2
10	7.15 ± .10	53 ± 9	1 ± 1	—12 ± 3

*Each value represents the mean and standard deviation of studies in 5 dogs.

four parameters; however, the rapidity and extent of the fall in oxygen tension suggest that anoxia was the primary cause of death (Modell, J. H., unpublished data).

Kristoffersen, Rattenborg, and Holaday[5] designed an experiment in dogs to separate the effects of hypoxia, hypercarbia, and acidosis during asphyxial death. In their dogs, death invariably resulted when the PaO_2 fell to 10 to 15 torr, whereas, hypercarbia without hypoxia was not fatal. When the tensions of arterial oxygen and carbon dioxide were kept normal, a fall in pHa to 6.50 was necessary to cause death of the animals.

Further evidence of the importance of hypoxia was given by Craig [6,7] who studied the breath-holding breaking point in human volunteers during simulated underwater swimming. He found the breath-holding breaking point to be 87 seconds at rest. The carbon dioxide tension of alveolar air ($PaCO_2$) was 51 torr and the tension of oxygen (PaO_2) was 73 torr. After hyperventilation, breath-holding could be maintained for 146 seconds. The $PaCO_2$, in this instance, only rose to 46 torr, whereas the PaO_2 dropped to 58 torr. When exercise followed hyperventilation, the breath-holding breaking point was 85 seconds. While the $PaCO_2$ was only 49 torr, the PaO_2 had dropped to 43 torr. He concluded that exercise, such as swimming, increased the metabolically produced carbon dioxide. Although $PaCO_2$ tended to rise, the rate of rise was limited because carbon dioxide stores had been depleted during hyperventilation. This, therefore, delayed the urge to breathe. With exercise, the oxygen tension fell to a level incompatible with cerebral function before the $PaCO_2$ became unbearable. Therefore, he concluded that loss of consciousness during underwater swimming was due to hypoxia, not to hypercarbia.

Redding and co-workers have also stressed the importance of hypoxia from airway obstruction.[8] They observed, in dogs, that the degree of saturation of hemoglobin in arterial blood with oxygen (SaO_2) was 10 perecent or less after 157 to 255 seconds of tracheal obstruction. They resuscitated their animals by intermittent positive pressure ventilation (IPPV). All of their dogs survived and after ten minutes of IPPV, their SaO_2 increased to at least 94 percent.

In treating 29 human victims of near-drowning, this author has seen two patients who probably suffered near-drowning without aspiration. In both cases, mouth-to-mouth resuscitation was given promptly at the scene of the accident. Spontaneous ventilation returned soon after the initiation of resuscitation and both patients had normal tensions for oxygen and carbon dioxide in arterial blood on admission to the hospital.

From all these data, it is safe to conclude that hypoxia is the single most important abnormality in death resulting from acute respiratory obstruction. It is well to remember, however, that the added effects of acidosis and hypercarbia may result in acceleration of the terminal event. If victims of *near-drowning without aspiration* are artificially ventilated before circulation ceases or irreversible central nervous system damage occurs, recovery will be dramatic and complete. If spontaneous ventilation begins while the patient is still in the water, however, aspiration will occur and a more complicated picture will be seen.

DROWNING AND NEAR-DROWNING WITH ASPIRATION

A recent study suggests that 85 percent of human drowning victims likely died from acute changes in blood gas tensions and acid-base balance.[9] While reliable blood gas and acid-base studies cannot be performed on drowning victims, data have been accumulated after near-drowning in humans [10-13] and under conditions simulating both near-drowning and drowning in animals.[1,8,14-24]

Oxygen

Changes in oxygenation have been measured in different ways. Some investigators have measured arterial oxygen tensions,[1,14-16] while others measured oxygen content [17-19] or the degree of saturation of hemoglobin with oxygen.[8,20-22] Man,[10-13] dogs,[1,8,14-19,22-24] sheep,[20,21] and rabbits [25] have been studied. Methods of simulating near-drowning and drowning differed slightly between the experimental studies. Some authors attempted to simulate near-downing by producing obstructive asphyxia prior to aspiration. Others introduced fluid directly into the trachea of spontaneously breathing animals. Regardless of the methods or species used all authors agreed that hypoxia occurred immediately after aspiration of fluid. Although the arterial oxygen tension was lower after total immersion than when small quantities of fluid were aspirated, profound changes occurred when as little as 1 to 3 ml/kg of water was aspirated.[14,15,20,21]

Unlike submersion without aspiration, when oxygenation returns to normal soon after resuscitation is started, the hypoxia seen

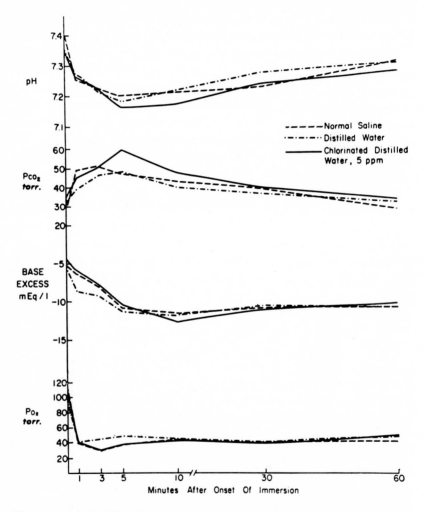

Figure 1. Arterial blood gas and acid-base changes subsequent to aspiration of 22 ml/kg of chlorinated distilled water, unchlorinated distilled water, and physiologic saline solution[1] (Reprinted with permission from *Anesthesiology*, *27*:33-41, 1966).

after aspiration of fluid is persistent. Figure 1 shows how arterial oxygen tension relates to other parameters of blood gas and acid-base balance after aspiration of 22 ml/kg of fresh water or normal saline solution. Although these animals were breathing spontaneously and hyperventilating when the 60-minute blood samples were drawn, significant arterial hypoxemia persisted throughout the experiment.[1] Even when smaller quantities of fresh water and sea water (11 ml/kg) were aspirated, arterial oxygen tension remained reduced for at least 72 hours following aspiration.[16] When animals which had aspirated equal quantities of distilled water and sea water were compared, the arterial oxygen tension was significantly lower one hour after sea water aspiration than after fresh water aspiration.[16] This suggests that, although hypoxia occurred after aspiration of either liquid, the etiology of the hypoxia might be different. Further consideration will be given to this hypothesis in Chapter IV.

Hypoxia has been reported consistently in human victims of near-drowning with aspiration.[10,11,13] Tables IV and V list the

TABLE IV

ARTERIAL BLOOD GAS AND pH VALUES FOUND ON ADMISSION TO THE HOSPITAL AFTER NEAR-DROWNING IN FRESH WATER

pHa	$PaCO_2$ (torr)	Base Excess (mEq/liter)	PaO_2 (torr)	$F_{1}O_2$
6.95*	64	—19	245	1.0
7.01	38	—22	28	.2
7.05*	59	—16	40	1.0 R
7.13	30	—19	67	.2
7.14	45	—14	68	.2
7.18	33	—15	110	1.0
7.19*	29	—16	108	±.8 R
7.21*	37	—13	175	1.0
7.22	54	— 7	123	1.0 R
7.28*	54	— 3	35	.4
7.33	41	— 4	127	1.0
7.40**	32	— 4	103	.2
7.44	32	— 2	76	.2
7.45**	35	1	84	.2

*These patients have been reported previously.[10]

**Patients likely did not aspirate fluid by clinical course

R = Ventilation supported mechanically

TABLE V

ARTERIAL BLOOD GAS AND pH VALUES FOUND ON ADMISSION TO THE
HOSPITAL AFTER NEAR-DROWNING IN SEA WATER

pHa	PaCO₂ (torr)	Base Excess (mEq/liter)	PaO₂ (torr)	FiO₂
7.03	36	—21	58	1.0
7.08	58	—14	21	1.0 R
7.20	46	—10	27	.2
7.29*	49	— 4	364	1.0 R
7.31	35	— 8	85	.8 R
7.35*	47	— 1	45	.2
7.46	25	— 5	71	.2
7.47	26	— 3	82	.4

*These patients have been reported previously.[10]

R = Ventilation supported mechanically

arterial blood gas changes observed within 60 minutes of immersion in 22 human near-drowning victims. In most cases, profound arterial hypoxemia was seen. The most severe was an arterial oxygen tension of 21 torr while the patient was being ventilated mechanically with 100 percent oxygen. Only two patients in this series had arterial oxygen tensions above 80 torr while they breathed room air. Both of these patients had been apneic when rescued, but began to breathe spontaneously soon after mouth-to-mouth ventilation was instituted. Their physical findings on admission to the hospital and subsequent clinical courses and blood gas determinations suggest that they did not actually aspirate fluid, but were victims of near-drowning without aspiration.

In many patients, a roentgenogram of the lungs shows evidence of fluid aspiration (Fig. 2.) However, severe hypoxia may be present without significant x-ray findings. Figure 3 shows the x-ray film of the chest of a child soon after he was admitted to the hospital. He had been apneic when rescued from a fresh water pool, and responded to artificial ventilation at the scene of the accident. The x-ray appears relatively normal, but his arterial oxygen tension was only 35 torr while he breathed 40% oxygen.

In some patients, the arterial oxygen tension returns to normal within forty-eight hours. Others, however, show persistent hypoxia for days and occassionally weeks following a near-drowning episode (see Chap. XIV). Relatively normal arterial oxygen tensions and alveolar-arterial oxygen gradients are frequently seen sooner when

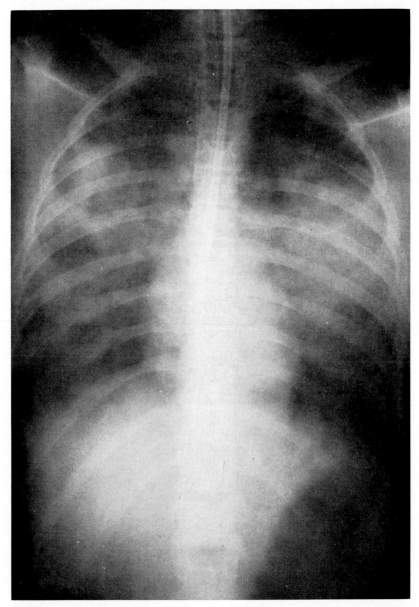

Figure 2. Chest x-ray of a patient taken two hours after resuscitation from near-drowning in chlorinated fresh water.

the patients breathe 100% oxygen than when they breathe room air.[10] A proposed mechanism for these observations is presented in Chapter IV.

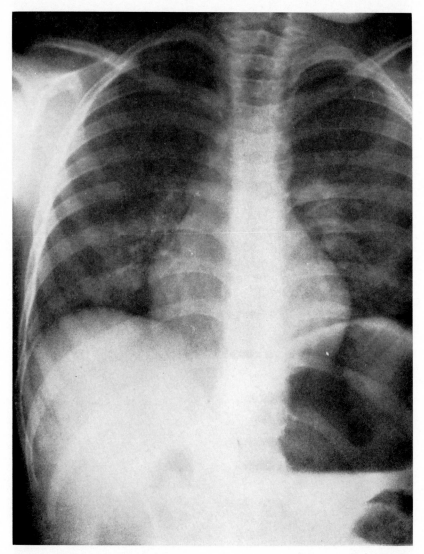

Figure 3. Chest x-ray of a patient one hour after near-drowning in chlorinated fresh water. At the time this x-ray was taken, the patient's PaO_2 was 35 torr while he breathed oxygen by mask[10] (Reprinted with permission from *JAMA, 203*:337-343, 1968).

Carbon Dioxide

The method of experimental study may influence the carbon dioxide changes seen after drowning. Although there is general agreement that after sea water aspiration the arterial carbon dioxide content and $PaCO_2$ increase,[14,17-19,22,24] conflicting data have been reported regarding carbon dioxide changes after fresh water aspiration. Austin *et al.*[24] have shown that the $PaCO_2$ decreases in dogs after they are totally immersed in fresh water. This is in conflict with the studies of Swann, which showed an initial increase in arterial carbon dioxide tension.[17-19] The difference between these two studies is that Swann's animals were awake and that they may have held their breath prior to aspiration. This would increase the carbon dioxide tension before the large quantities of aspirated fluid diluted the carbon dioxide in the blood.

When carbon dioxide tension was studied in anesthetized dogs after near-drowning,[1,15] three minutes after fresh water aspiration there was an increase in $PaCO_2$. As larger quantities of fresh water were aspirated, however, the values reached a plateau. Under con-

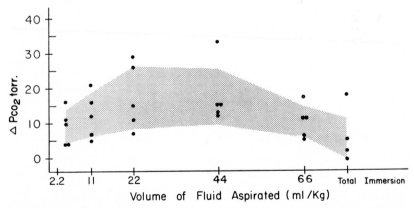

Figure 4. Changes in $PaCO_2$ three minutes post-aspiration of fresh water are plotted as a function of the quantity of water aspirated. Values are plotted as change from preaspiration levels for each animal. Standard deviation for each group is shaded to more clearly visualize trends[15] (Reprinted with permission from *Anesthesiology, 27*:662-672, 1966).

ditions of total immersion, the rise in $PaCO_2$ was insignificant (Fig. 4). These studies support the hypothesis that the carbon dioxide changes after aspiration of large quantities of hypotonic fluid are limited by the dilutional effect that occurs when the water is absorbed into the vascular space. The influence of time after aspiration of 22 ml/kg of fresh water (with or without chlorine) or normal saline on $PaCO_2$ is seen in Figure 1. There was a rapid increase in $PaCO_2$, followed by a decrease to normal values as the animals spontaneously began to hyperventilate.

The arterial carbon dioxide tension varies considerably in human near-drowning victims (Tables IV and V). There does not seem to be any barrier to the elimination of carbon dioxide since the $PaCO_2$ was below 50 torr in more than 75 percent of the patients listed. The higher values found in five of these patients suggest hypoventilation at the time the blood samples were drawn. No difficulty was encountered in blowing off the $PaCO_2$ in any of these patients when ventilation was subsequently assisted or controlled with mechanical devices. These data agree with those of Hasan et al., who reported a mean $PaCO_2$ of 41 ± S.D. 12 torr in 32 victims of near-drowning.[13]

Acid-Base Changes

In animals, the pH decreased following aspiration, regardless of the kind of water aspirated or the technique of study.[1,14-19,24] The changes may be transient following aspiration of small quantities of fluid, but following total immersion there was a progressive fall in pH with the passage of time.[14,15,24] Immediately after aspiration, a combined metabolic and respiratory acidosis was seen as both a base deficit and a rise in $PaCO_2$ occurred.[11]

Austin et al.[24] reported that the bicarbonate concentration decreased in dogs after total immersion in fresh water and temporarily increased after total immersion in sea water. This can be attributed, in part, to the dramatic changes in circulating blood volume which can occur after aspiration of hypo- or hypertonic fluids. If sublethal quantities of fluid were aspirated, the animals began to hyperventilate and eliminate carbon dioxide. However, a significant base deficit, presumably related to the persistent hypoxemia, was still observed one hour after aspiration.[1] This observation, and the fact that lactic acid increased in excess of pyruvate after drowning,[24] indicates that metabolic acidosis persists.

In a series of patients studied by this author, acidosis (pH$\leq$

7.35) was seen in 78 percent of near-drowning victims when pH was measured soon after rescue (Tables IV and V). The acidosis was respiratory in two patients ($PaCO_2 \gtreqqless 46$ torr), metabolic in nine patients (base deficit $\gtreqqless 4$ mEp/1), and a combination of respiratory and metabolic in six. Two additional patients had metabolic acidosis, but the pH was returned to normal by compensatory hyperventilation. Hasan *et al.* report similar findings in 32 near-drowning victims. Sixty percent of their patients had a metabolic acidosis and 21 percent had a combined metabolic and respiratory acidosis.[13] In both series, sodium bicarbonate or buffers were administered immediately when a base deficit was found. Thus, persistent metabolic acidosis was not seen. In cases where blood gases have not been measured until later in the hospital course, metabolic acidosis has been reported late during recovery of humans from near-drowning.[12,26,27]

Summary

The magnitude of changes in arterial blood gas tensions and acid-base balance is somewhat dependent upon whether they are studied after near-drowning or drowning by total immersion. Acute asphyxia occurs in all, however; and, while $PaCO_2$ may return to normal spontaneously, arterial hypoxemia and a metabolic acidosis persist unless treated after near-drowning with aspiration. Hypoxemia is sometimes evident while the patient breathes room air even after the alveolar-arterial oxygen gradient, measured while breathing 100% oxygen, is no longer significant. This, plus the fact that the degree of hypoxia is greater after aspiration of sea water than after an equal quantity of fresh water, suggests the possibility of a multiple etiology for the hypoxia of near-drowning.

REFERENCES

1. Modell, J. H.; Gaub, M.; Moya, F.; Vestal, B., and Swarz, H.: Physiologic effects of near drowning with chlorinated fresh water, distilled water and isotonic saline. *Anesthesiology, 27*:33-41, 1966.
2. Coryllos, P. N.: Mechanical resuscitation in advanced forms of asphyxia. A clinical and experimental study in the different methods of resuscitation. *Surg Gynec Obstet, 66*:698-722, 1938.
3. Lougheed, D. W.; Janes, J. M., and Hall, G. E.: Physiological studies in experimental asphyxia and drowning. *Canad Med Ass J, 40*:423-428, 1939.

4. Cot, C.: *Les Asphyxies Accidentelles* (submersion, electrocution, intoxication oxycarbonique). Etude clinique, therapeutique et preventive. Paris, Editions medicales N. Maloine, 1931.

5. Kristoffersen, M. B.; Rattenborg, C. C., and Holaday, D. A.: Asphyxial death: the roles of acute anoxia, hypercarbia and acidosis. *Anesthesiology, 28*:488-497, 1967.

6. Craig, A. B., Jr.: Underwater swimming and loss of consciousness. *JAMA, 176*:255-258, 1961.

7. Craig, A. B., Jr.: Causes of loss of consciousness during underwater swimming. *J Appl Physiol, 16*:583-586, 1961.

8. Redding, J.; Voigt, G. C., and Safar, P.: Drowning treated with intermittent positive pressure breathing. *J Appl Physiol, 15*:849-854, 1960.

9. Modell, J. H., and Davis, J. H.: Electrolyte changes in human drowning victims. *Anesthesiology, 30*:414-420, 1969.

10. Modell, J. H.; Davis, J. H.; Giammona, S. T.; Moya, F., and Mann, J. B.: Blood gas and electrolyte changes in human near-drowning victims. JAMA, *203*:337-343, 1968.

11. Modell, J. H.: Ventilation/perfusion changes during mechanical ventilation. *Dis Chest, 55*:447-451, 1969.

12. Warden, J. C.: Respiratory insufficiency following near-drowning in sea water. *JAMA, 201*:887-890, 1967.

13. Hasan, S.; Avery, W. G.; Fabian, C., and Sackner, M. A.: Near drowning in humans. A report of 36 patients. *Chest, 59*:191-197, 1971.

14. Modell, J. H.; Moya, F.; Newby, E. J.; Ruiz, B. C., and Showers, A. V.: The effects of fluid volume in seawater drowning. *Ann Intern Med, 67*:68-80, 1967.

15. Modell, J. H., and Moya, F.: Effects of volume of aspirated fluid during chlorinated fresh water drowning. *Anesthesiology, 27*:662-672, 1966.

16. Modell, J. H.; Moya, F.; Williams, H. D., and Weibley, T. C.: Changes in blood gases and A-aDO$_2$ during near-drowning. *Anesthesiology, 29*:456-465, 1968.

17. Swann, H. G., and Spafford, N. R.: Body salt and water changes during fresh and sea water drowning. *Texas Rep Biol Med, 9*:356-382, 1951.

18. Swann, H. G., and Brucer, M.: The cardiorespiratory and biochemical events during rapid anoxic death. VI. Fresh water and sea water drowning. *Texas Rep Biol Med, 7*:604-618, 1949.

19. Swann, H. G.; Brucer, M.; Moore, C., and Vezien, B. L.: Fresh water and sea water drowning: A study of the terminal cardiac and biochemical events. *Texas Rep Biol Med, 5*:423-437, 1947.

20. Halmagyi, D. F. J., and Colebatch, H. J. H.: Ventilation and circulation after fluid aspiration. *J Appl Physiol, 16*:35-40, 1961.

21. Colebatch, H. J. H., and Halmagyi, D. F. J.: Lung mechanics and resuscitation after fluid aspiration. *J Appl Physiol, 16*:684-696, 1961.

22. Redding, J. S.; Voigt, G. C., and Safar, P.: Treatment of sea-water aspiration. *J Appl Physiol, 15*:1113-1116, 1960.

23. Farthmann, E. H., and Davidson, A. I. G.: Fresh water drowning at lowered body temperature; an experimental study. *Amer J Surg, 109*:410-415, 1965.
24. Austin, W. H.; Stinebaugh, B. J.; Rand, P. W., and Lacombe, E.: The effects of drowning on acid-base balance. *J Maine Med Ass, 58*:20-23, 1967.
25. Modell, J. H.; Weibley, T. C.; Ruiz, B. C., and Newby, E. J.: Serum electrolyte concentrations after fresh-water aspiration: a comparison of species. *Anesthesiology, 30*:421-425, 1969.
26. Ohlsson, K., and Beckman, M.: Drowning—reflections based on two cases. *Acta Chir Scand, 128*:327-339, 1964.
27. King, R. B., and Webster, I. W.: A case of recovery from drowning and prolonged anoxia. *Med J Aust, 1*:919-920, 1964.

Chapter IV

PULMONARY EFFECTS

IT HAS BEEN SHOWN, in the preceding chapter, that hypoxemia is the most consistent finding following near-drowning. While many factors play a role in the development of hypoxemia, its magnitude is more severe following aspiration of sea water than following aspiration of an equal quantity of fresh water.[1] This suggests, that, although hypoxemia occurs with aspiration of either type of fluid, its etiology may be different. If treatment is to be aimed at the specific pathophysiologic processes involved, it is important to understand the etiology of this hypoxemia. This chapter will review the experimental data obtained in animals and relate them to observations made in human near-drowning victims.

Karpovich[2] suggested that water in the alveoli and conducting airways blocked ventilation and subsequent resuscitation. Since his studies in 1933, other investigators have demonstrated that aspiration of sea water leads to an increase in volume of fluid within the airspaces in the lung.[3,4] For example, Halmagyi showed that the weight of the lungs of rats increased by three times the amount of sea water aspirated.[5] If one attempts to drain the lungs of dogs by gravity or mechanical suction after sea water aspiration, more fluid is harvested than was originally poured into the trachea.[3,4] On the other hand, after fresh water aspiration, the lungs of rats did not increase in weight.[5] When a sublethal quantity of fresh water was instilled into the trachea of anesthetized dogs, it was absorbed so rapidly that after only three minutes significant amounts of water could not be recovered from the airway.[1,6,7]

Since sea water draws fluid or plasma into the alveoli, it is easy to understand why pulmonary edema occurs in patients suffering from near-drowning in sea water. Evidence of pulmonary edema by direct observation of frothy fluid, auscultation of rales, or findings on chest x-rays is also reported after fresh water near-drowning.[8-24]

Since water cannot be drained from the lungs after fresh water aspiration, other mechanisms are necessary to explain these findings. It has been suggested that pulmonary edema after fresh water aspiration is due to overloading of the circulation by absorbed fluid and subsequent congestive heart failure.[25] This explanation, although reasonable when large volumes of water are aspirated, cannot account for the pulmonary edema seen after aspiration of small quantities of fresh water.

Some insight into this problem can be gained from studies on the effect of aspirated water on the surface tension properties of pulmonary surfactant.[26] Pulmonary surfactant extracted from the lungs of animals which died while totally immersed in fresh water showed abnormal surface tension values (Table VI). In contrast, during total immersion in isotonic saline solution or in sea water, some normal pulmonary surfactant was washed from the lungs with respiratory movements. However, sufficient quantities of surfactant remained so that the material extracted from the lung at autopsy displayed surface tension properties compatible with normal pulmonary surfactant. It is known that alveoli which are deficient in normal surfactant are unstable and prone to collapse. In addition, such alveoli frequently leak fluid. It is likely, therefore, that the pulmonary edema which occurs after sea water aspiration is due, primarily, to an osmotic gradient across the alveolar capillary membrane with an accumulation of fluid in the alveoli. After fresh water aspiration, however, loss of normal surface tension activity of pulmonary surfactant leads to alveolar instability and development of pulmonary edema.

Some authors have observed that it requires high pressures to ventilate patients immediately after aspiration of liquid.[9] Halmagyi and Colebatch [27-30] demonstrated in sheep that aspiration of as little as 1 ml/kg of water caused a significant fall in lung compliance. Vagotomy[30] and administration of either atropine or isoproterenol[29] decreased the degree of change in compliance after aspiration. From these findings, they concluded that aspiration of water triggers a parasympathetic reflex, producing airway closure.[29] The author and his colleagues[1] demonstrated an increase in arterial oxygen tension and a decrease in intrapulmonary shunt or venous admixture when high concentrations of isoproterenol were administered intravenously to dogs after aspiration of either fresh water or sea water. This effect was only temporary, however, and although isopro-

TABLE VI

SURFACE TENSION ACTIVITY (DYNES/CM) OF PULMONARY SURFACTANT AND
TRACHEAL FLUID FROM DOGS AFTER TOTAL IMMERSION

	Lung Extracts		Tracheal Fluid	
	Min. S.T. - Max. S.T.		Min. S.T. - Max. S.T.	
Type of Water	@ 20 cm²	@ 100 cm²	@ 20 cm²	@ 100 cm²
Fresh	21 ± 6	58 ± 9	30 ± 3	54 ± 5
Chlorinated fresh	19 ± 4	49 ± 4	27 ± 4	58 ± 3
Saline (0.9%)	9 ± 3	56 ± 7	5 ± 3	63 ± 7
Sea	7 ± 4	45 ± 9	7 ± 4	46 ± 9

Modified with permission from *Amer J Dis Child, 114*:612-616, 1967.

terenol infusion was continued, the improvement in oxygenation did not persist. This suggests that another process was present and, therefore, it is unlikely that reflex airway closure is the predominant factor causing persistent arterial hypoxemia.

Immediately after aspiration of either fresh water or sea water, a large alveolar-arterial oxygen gradient is seen during the breathing of 100% oxygen. This suggests that hypoxia after near-drowning is predominantly due to absolute intrapulmonary shunting, i.e. perfusion of nonventilated alveoli.[1] The total shunt measured during the breathing of air is significantly greater than that measured while breathing 100% oxygen one hour after fresh water aspiration. Thus, in addition to the absolute shunt seen following aspiration of either fresh or sea water, a relative shunt due to ventilation-perfusion imbalance and/or diffusion abnormalities also plays a role in the hypoxia seen after fresh water aspiration.

Periodic hyperinflation of the lungs after aspiration of fresh water produced a significant, lasting increase in arterial oxygen tension and a decrease in shunt, but deliberate hyperinflation had no significant lasting effect on these parameters after aspiration of an equal quantity of sea water.[1,30] A further beneficial effect of hyperinflation after fresh water aspiration also can be seen since compliance increases.[30] These findings further support the hypothesis that, although hypoxia occurs after aspiration of either fluid, the mechanism is different. The evidence points toward a space occupying lesion in the alveoli after sea water aspiration (fluid-filled). After fresh water aspiration, however, alveolar collapse, or atelectasis, due to surfactant changes is likely the single most important cause of hypoxia.

FACTORS CONTRIBUTING TO HYPOXIA IN NEAR-DROWNING

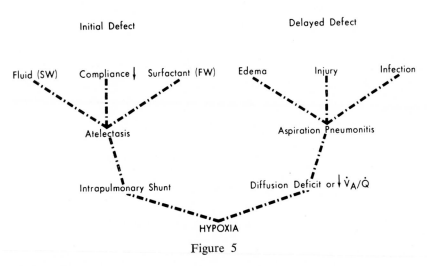

Figure 5

During recovery from aspiration of both fresh and sea water, significant hypoxia is seen during breathing of room air, even after the alveolar-arterial oxygen gradient while breathing 100% oxygen has returnd to normal.[1,31] This suggests that areas of non-uniform ventilation or diffusion problems cause hypoxia even after the absolute intrapulmonary shunt is no longer of clinical significance (Fig. 5). A number of changes which occur following aspiration of fluid could contribute to this delayed defect. Organization of the proteinaceous exudate formed during pulmonary edema may lead to formation of layers resembling hyaline membranes. The injury to the alveolar-capillary membrane, caused by aspirated hypotonic or hypertonic fluid, leads to changes in the alveolar architecture. In addition, many of these patients develop secondary infections of the lung.

A variety of microscopic findings have been reported after fluid aspiration. The lungs of rats which aspirated small quantities of fresh water (0.1 ml/100 mg body weight) did not show changes when studied by electron microscopy. After aspiration of the same small quantity of sea water, however, increases in lung weight and intra-alveolar hemorrhages were observed.[5] On the other hand, if the lungs of rats were perfused via the trachea with large quantities of fresh water, there was a widening of the alveolar septae, a collapse of the capillaries, a decrease in the number of red blood cells, an enlargement of the endothelial and septae cell nuclei, a swelling of the mitochrondria, and obliteration of the cell outlines. Presumably, these changes all can be attributed to rapid absorption of large quantities of fresh water from the alveoli. When rat lungs were perfused intratracheally with sea water, changes were less marked and the septal and endothelial nuclei were small and dark. Red blood cells frequently were seen in the capillaries, and although there was irregular folding of cell walls, the overall architecture of the lung was preserved.[32] The irregular walls and shrinkage of the cells that was seen probably results from the movement of fluid from the tissue into the alveoli filled with sea water. Thus, the microscopic changes which occur are different when very small or very large quantities of water are aspirated. This may account for some of the differences reported in humans who are autopsied after they drown. In any event, pathologic changes can occur in the alveoli from aspiration of either hypo- or hypertonic fluid.

Another frequent finding on autopsy in both humans and animals soon after death by drowning is hyperexpansion of the lungs with areas resembling acute emphysema.[15,20,33] This could represent rupture of alveoli from the wide fluctuation in airway pressure generated during violent ventilatory efforts against a closed glottis, or obstruction from a column of water in the airway during submersion. If the patient survives for at least twelve hours after near-drowning, only to die later, the lungs will frequently show evidence of bronchopneumonia, multiple abscesses, mechanical injury, and deposition of hyaline material in the alveoli from approximately twelve hours to the third day.[15] These findings are not surprising in light of the fact that Fuller[10] reported that 70 percent of humans autopsied after drowning showed evidence of aspirating something other than water, e.g. vomitus, mud, sand, or algae. In spite of the severe changes in pulmonary function which can occur during the acute near-drowning episode, Butt *et al.*[34] were unable to demonstrate any consistent pattern of abnormality in pulmonary function or arterial oxygenation in 13 patients who were studied after recovery from near-drowning. It seems, therefore, that these acute changes are completely reversible.

Summary

It appears that the initial cause of hypoxemia after near-drowning is shunting of blood through perfused, but nonventilated, alveoli (Fig. 5). The underlying mechanism for nonventilation of alveoli after aspiration of fresh water is an alteration of the normal surface tension properties of pulmonary surfactant with a collapse of the alveoli. Unless the surface active material is regenerated, uneven ventilation and recurrent collapse of alveoli occur; even after they have been forcibly reinflated. After aspiration of sea water, fluid in the alveoli prevents ventilation. In addition, a decrease in compliance and an increase in airway resistance also contribute to the hypoxemia seen.

Once a true or absolute intrapulmonary shunt can no longer be demonstrated when patients or animals are allowed to breath 100% oxygen, hypoxemia frequently persists while they breathe room air. This suggests that a delayed defect exists due to abnormal ventilation-perfusion ratios and/or a diffusion deficit. Likely, this delayed lesion is the result of aspiration pneumonitis and its accompanying pulmonary edema, damage to the alveolar capillary membrane from the hyper- or hypotonicity of the water, and secondary infection.

REFERENCES

1. Modell, J. H.; Moya, F.; Williams, H. D., and Weibley, T. C.: Changes in blood gases and A-aDO$_2$ during near-drowning. *Anesthesiology, 29*:456-465, 1968.
2. Karpovich, P. V.: Water in the lungs of drowned animals. *Arch Path (Chicago), 15*:828-833, 1933.
3. Modell, J. H.; Moya, F.; Newby, E. J.; Ruiz, B. C., and Showers, A. V.: The effects of fluid volume in seawater drowning. *Ann Intern Med, 67*:68-80, 1967.
4. Redding, J. S.; Voigt, G. C., and Safar, P.: Treatment of sea-water aspiration. *J Appl Physiol, 15*:1113-1116, 1960.
5. Halmagyi, D. F. J.: Lung changes and incidence of respiratory arrest in

rats after aspiration of sea and fresh water. *J Appl Physiol, 16*:41-44, 1961.

6. Redding, J.; Voigt, G. C., and Safar, P.: Drowning treated with intermittent positive pressure breathing. *J Appl Physiol, 15*:849-854, 1960.

7. Modell, J. H., and Moya, F.: Effects of volume of aspirated fluid during chlorinated fresh water drowning. *Anesthesiology, 27*:662-672, 1966.

8. Cahill, J. M.: Drowning: the problem of nonfatal submersion and the unconscious patient. *Surg Clin N Amer, 48*:423-430, 1968.

9. Warden, J. C.: Respiratory insufficiency following near-drowning in sea water. *JAMA, 201*:887-890, 1967.

10. Fuller, R. H.: The clinical pathology of human near-drowning. *Proc Roy Soc Med, 56*:33-38, 1963.

11. Romagosa, J. J.; Menville, L. J., and Leckert, J. T.: Radiographic changes in the lungs during recovery from drowning. *Radiology, 55*:517-521, 1950.

12. Modell, J. H.: Resuscitation after aspiration of chlorinated fresh water. *JAMA, 185*:651-655, 1963.

13. Saline, M., and Baum, G. L.: The submersion syndrome. *Ann Intern Med, 41*:1134-1138, 1954.

14. Dumitru, A. P., and Hamilton, F. G.: A mechanism of drowning. *Anesth Analg (Cleveland), 42*:170-176, 1963.

15. Fuller, R. H.: The 1962 Wellcome prize essay. Drowning and the post-immersion syndrome. A clinicopathologic study. *Milit Med, 128*:22-36, 1963.

16. Fainer, D. C.: Near drowning in sea water and fresh water. *Ann Intern Med, 59*:537-541, 1963.

17. Griffin, G. E.: Near-drowning: Its pathophysiology and treatment in man. *Milit Med, 131*:12-21, 1966.

18. Kvittingen, T. D., and Naess, A.: Recovery from drowning in fresh water. *Brit Med J, 5341*:1315-1317, 1963.

19. Wong, F. M., and Grace, W. J.: Sudden death after near-drowning. *JAMA, 186*:724-726, 1963.

20. Imburg, J., and Hartney, T. C.: Drowning and the treatment of non-fatal submersion: I. Drowning and non-fatal submersion laboratory studies and human data. *Pediatrics, 37*:684-698, 1966.

21. Munroe, W. D.: Hemoglobinuria from near-drowning. *J Pediat, 64*:57-62, 1964.

22. Rosenbaum, H. T.; Thompson, W. L., and Fuller, R. H.: Radiographic pulmonary changes in near-drowning. *Radiology, 83*:306-313, 1964.

23. Haddy, T. B., and Disenhouse, R. B.: Acute pulmonary edema due to near-drowning in fresh water. *J Pediat, 44*:565-569, 1954.

24. Swann, Jr., H. G.: Occurrence of pulmonary edema in sudden asphyxial deaths. *AMA Arch Path, 69*:557-570, 1960.

25. Swann, H. G., and Spafford, N. R.: Body salt and water changes during fresh and sea water drowning. *Texas Rep Biol Med, 9*:356-382, 1951.

26. Giammona, S. T., and Modell, J. H.: Drowning by total immersion. Effects on pulmonary surfactant of distilled water, isotonic saline and sea water. *Amer J Dis Child, 114*:612-616, 1967.
27. Halmagyi, D. F. J., and Colebatch, H. J. H.: The drowned lung. A physiological approach to its mechanism and management. *Aust Ann Med, 10*:68-77, 1961.
28. Colebatch, H. J. H., and Halmagyi, D. F. J.: Reflex pulmonary hypertension of fresh water aspiration. *J Appl Physiol, 18*:179-185, 1963.
29. Colebatch, H. J. H., and Halmagyi, D. F. J.: Reflex airway reaction to fluid aspiration. *J Appl Physiol, 17*:787-794, 1962.
30. Colebatch, H. J. H., and Halmagyi, D. F. J.: Lung mechanics and resuscitation after fluid aspiration. *J Appl Physiol, 16*:684-696, 1961.
31. Modell, J. H.; Davis, J. H.; Giammona, S. T.; Moya, F., and Mann, J. B.: Blood gas and electrolyte changes in human near-drowning victims. *JAMA, 203*:337-343, 1968.
32. Reidbord, H. E., and Spitz, W. U.: Ultrastructural alterations in rat lungs. Changes after intratracheal perfusion with freshwater and seawater. *Arch Path, 81*:103-111, 1966.
33. Miloslavich, E. L.: Pathological anatomy of death by drowning. *Amer J Clin Path, 4*:42-49, 1934.
34. Butt, M. P.; Jalowayski, A.; Modell, J. H., and Giammona, S. T.: Pulmonary function after resuscitation from near-drowning. *Anesthesiology, 32*:275-277, 1970.

Chapter V

BLOOD VOLUME

T HE DIRECTION AND MAGNITUDE of changes in blood volume after drowning and near-drowning are dependent upon both the tonicity and the volume of water aspirated.

FRESH WATER DROWNING AND NEAR-DROWNING

Fresh water, being hypotonic, is absorbed rapidly from the lungs into the circulation. Within minutes of aspiration, fresh water could not be recovered from the trachea of experimental animals.[1-4] When small quantities of water (2.2 ml/kg) were aspirated, there was no significant increase in blood volume. However, a significant hypervolemia occurred within two to three minutes if dogs aspirated 11 ml/kg or more of fresh water.[1,3] Three minutes after aspiration, there was a linear relationship between the volume of fluid aspirated and the increase in blood volume. The blood volume increased by 1.4 percent for every milliliter per kilogram of water aspirated, until more than 44 ml/kg body weight of water was aspirated (Fig. 6). At this level, the blood volume reached a plateau. This plateau corresponded to the volume of water aspirated when 80 percent of the dogs died acutely of ventricular fibrillation.[1] It is likely that cessation of circulation limited the increase in blood volume above this level.

The influx of hypotonic fluid into the circulation immediately after drowning by total immersion in fresh water also can be reflected in a decrease in osmolarity and viscosity of blood.[5] The dramatic effect on blood density can be seen in Figure 7, which is taken from the classical studies of Swann et al.[6]

This increase in circulating blood volume is also compatible with the elevation of central venous pressure that occurs after aspiration of fresh water.[4,7] Within approximately 15 minutes of aspiration, however, the central venous pressure approached normal in

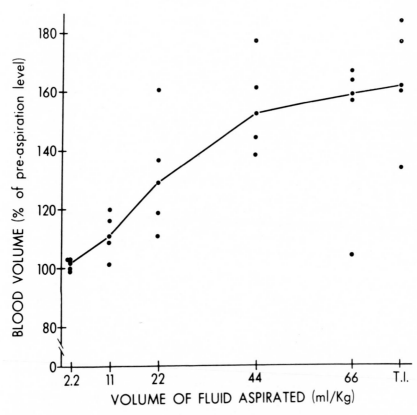

Figure 6. Blood volume three minutes after aspiration of fresh water. The percent change in blood volume is plotted as a function of the quantity of water aspirated. Each point represents change from preaspiration value for the individual animal (Reprinted with permission from *Anesthesiology, 27*: 662-672, 1966).

animals that survived fresh water near-drowning.[4] This suggests that, although hypervolemia occurred immediately following aspiration of fresh water, it was transient. In further support of this hypothesis, it has been shown that a significant increase in blood volume occurred three minutes after dogs aspirated 11 ml/kg of fresh water.[1] Yet, one hour later, the blood volume returned to its preaspiration level (Modell, unpublished data). This readjustment in blood volume was probably due to the redistribution of the fluid into other body compartments and to transudation of plasma into the lung.[3,8]

Reports of blood volume determinations in humans after fresh water aspiration are scarce. In one case, reported by Fuller, a significant deficit in plasma volume was seen. The time at which the studies were done relative to the time of near-drowning was not reported, however. On the basis of hemoglobin and hematocrit levels in this and other patients, he concluded that fresh water near-drowning victims frequently show hemoconcentration, and they may require plasma replacement.[8] The possible limitations of using hemoglobin and hematocrit concentrations to evaluate blood volume after fresh water near-drowning are discussed in Chapter VII.

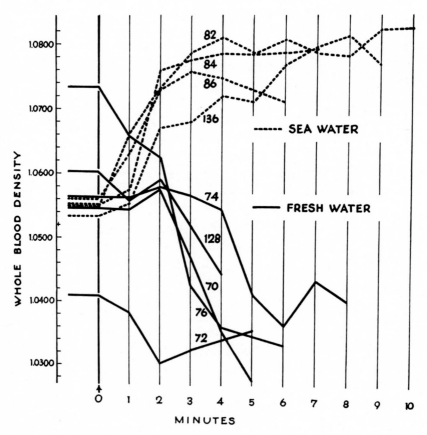

Figure 7. Changes in blood density during drowning (Reprinted with permission from *Tex Rep Biol Med,* 5:423-437, 1947).

SEA WATER DROWNING AND NEAR-DROWNING

A few minutes after sea water is aspirated, more fluid can be recovered from the trachea than was originally instilled. This is in striking contrast to what follows aspiration of fresh water. This is due to the hypertonicity of the sea water, which draws plasma from the circulation into the lung. The actual transfer of plasma water into the airway was confirmed in dogs by Swann.[3] He found deuterium oxide in the tracheal fluid after sea water drowning, when it had been injected into the circulation. The loss of albumin into the lungs of dogs has also been demonstrated after sea water aspiration. Three minutes after total immersion in sea water, approximately 7 percent of an intravenous dose of radio-iodinated serum albumin RISA (^{131}I) was found in the tracheal fluid.[9]

Aspiration of 2.2 ml/kg of sea water produced no immediate effect on blood volume in dogs, but a decrease of approximately 5 percent occurred within one hour. When at least 11 ml/kg was aspirated, a significant decrease in blood volume occurred within one minute.[3,9] The change in blood volume seen after sea water aspiration was inversely proportional to the quantity of fluid aspirated. While the increase in blood volume seen after fresh water near-drowning was transient, the hypovolemia seen after sea water aspiration can persist for forty-eight hours.[10] Redding, Voigt, and Safar[11] have demonstrated the importance of plasma replacement upon improving survival rate of dogs during resuscitation from sea water near-drowning.

As might be expected, there is an increase in both osmolarity and viscosity after sea water drowning.[5] The effect of drowning by total immersion in sea water on blood density is shown in Figure 7.[6]

Due to the loss of albumin from the circulation, it is particularly difficult to quantitate changes in blood volume with radioactive albumin tracers (RISA) after sea water aspiration. The effect of this loss is shown in Figure 8, where blood volume was measured one, three, and ten minutes after sea water aspiration using a single dose of tracer which was injected immediately prior to aspiration.[9] The approximate slope of the albumin decay curve can be seen in Figure 9, where blood volume measured with a single tracer injection is plotted against time after total immersion in sea water. On the surface, these results can be interpreted to mean that an

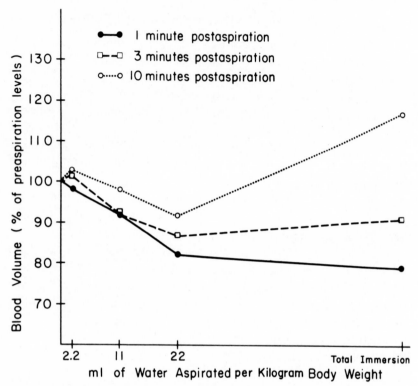

Figure 8. Changes in blood volume one, three, and ten minutes after sea water aspiration as measured with RISA (^{131}I) (Reprinted with permission from *Ann Intern Med*, 67:68-80, 1967).

increase in blood volume occurred ten minutes after total immersion in sea water. When blood volume was determined with ^{51}Cr tagged red blood cells, different results were obtained.

Although there is a decrease in the size of red blood cells after sea water drowning, they are not lost from the circulation. The ^{51}Cr tagged red blood cell technique is, therefore, a more accurate method for blood volume determinations in this instance than the RISA technique. With the ^{51}Cr, the average blood volume ten minutes after total immersion in sea water was shown, in dogs, to be 74 percent of the preaspiration level.[9]

Although the hemoglobin and hematocrit values are frequently compatible with a decrease in blood volume after sea water aspiration, they usually do not reflect hypervolemia after fresh water

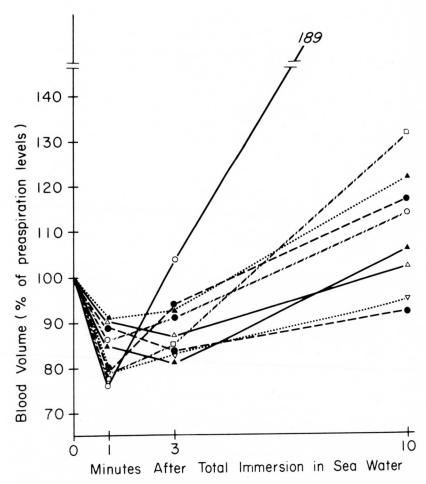

Figure 9. Changes in blood volume after total immersion in sea water as measured with RISA (^{125}I or ^{131}I). Each line represents the values found in an individual animal (Reprinted with permission from *Ann Intern Med, 67*: 68-80, 1967).

near-drowning.[1,4,9] Individual variations may occur, however, and caution should be used in extrapolating from hemoglobin and hematocrit levels to blood volume.

Summary

The changes in blood volume which occur after aspiration of fluid are dependent upon both the tonicity and the volume of fluid aspirated. After fresh water near-drowning and drowning, there is an immediate increase in blood volume due to the rapid transfer of the hypotonic fluid into the circulation. In those who survive (both animals and humans), this hypervolemia is transient. After sea water aspiration, the blood volume decreases; again, the degree is proportional to the quantity of fluid aspirated. Since all patients do not aspirate the same quantity of fluid, no general predictions of blood volume changes can be made when evaluating a specific near-drowning victim.

REFERENCES

1. Modell, J. H., and Moya, F.: Effects of volume of aspirated fluid during chlorinated fresh water drowning. *Anesthesiology, 27*:662-672, 1966.
2. Starzecki, B., and Halmagyi, D. F. J.: Absorption of inhaled water in experimental pulmonary edema and embolism. *Amer J Physiol, 201*: 762-764, 1961.
3. Swann, H. G., and Spafford, N. R.: Body salt and water changes during fresh and sea water drowning. *Texas Rep Biol Med, 9*:356-382, 1951.
4. Modell, J. H.; Gaub, M.; Moya, F.; Vestal, B., and Swarz, H.: Physiologic effects of near drowning with chlorinated fresh water, distilled water and isotonic saline. *Anesthesiology, 27*:33-41, 1966.
5. Rand, P. W.; Lacombe, E.; Austin, W. H., and Stinebaugh, B. J.: The effects of drowning on blood viscosity. *J Maine Med Ass, 58*:23-27, 1967.
6. Swann, H. G.; Brucer, M.; Moore, C., and Vezien, B. L.: Fresh water and sea water drowning: A study of the terminal cardiac and biochemical events. *Texas Rep Biol Med, 5*:423-437, 1947.
7. Spitz, W. U., and Blanke, R. V.: Mechanism of death in fresh-water drowning. I. An experimental approach to the problem. *Arch Path (Chicago), 71*:661-668, 1961.
8. Fuller, R. H.: The 1962 Wellcome prize essay. Drowning and the post-immersion syndrome. A clinicopathologic study. *Milit Med, 128*:22-36, 1963.
9. Modell, J. H.; Moya, F.; Newby, E. J.; Ruiz, B. C., and Showers, A. V.: The effects of fluid volume in seawater drowning. *Ann Intern Med, 67*:68-80, 1967.
10. Modell, J. H.; Moya, F.; Williams, H. D., and Weibley, T. C.: Changes in blood gases and A-aDO$_2$ during near-drowning. *Anesthesiology, 29*:456-465, 1968.
11. Redding, J. S.; Voigt, G. C., and Safar, P.: Treatment of sea-water aspiration. *J Appl Physiol, 15*:1113-1116, 1960.

Chapter VI

SERUM ELECTROLYTE CHANGES

T HE CHANGES IN SERUM electrolyte concentrations which occur following drowning and near-drowning are dependent upon both the type and the volume of water aspirated. If the victim survives near-drowning, the electrolyte changes are likely to be transient and spontaneously revert to normal.

FRESH WATER

It was suggested in the nineteenth century by Devergie and confirmed by Revenstorf[1] in 1902 that hypotonic fluid appeared in the circulation after it was aspirated. Modell and Moya have shown that within three minutes of aspiration, there was a 1.4 percent increase in circulating blood volume for each milliliter of distilled water aspirated per kilogram body weight.[2] This influx of water into the blood diluted the extracellular electrolytes. While no significant changes in serum sodium, chloride, and calcium concentrations were found three minutes postaspiration when dogs aspirated small quantities of fluid (11 ml/kg or less), when they aspirated 22 ml/kg or more a significant reduction in concentration of these electrolytes occurred. The resulting levels were inversely proportional to the volume of fluid aspirated[2] (Fig. 10).

The changes in serum potassium concentration three minutes after aspiration of 11 ml/kg or less of fresh water were not significant. However, dogs did show a significant increase in serum potassium when they aspirated at least 22 ml/kg of fluid.[2] While some hemolysis of red blood cells takes place after aspiration of this quantity of fresh water (see Chap. VII), the potassium concentration in the red cells of the dog[3] is only 10 mEq/liter. Thus, it is unlikely that hemolysis, alone, is responsible for this increase. The acute severe hypoxia and acidosis which are characteristic of

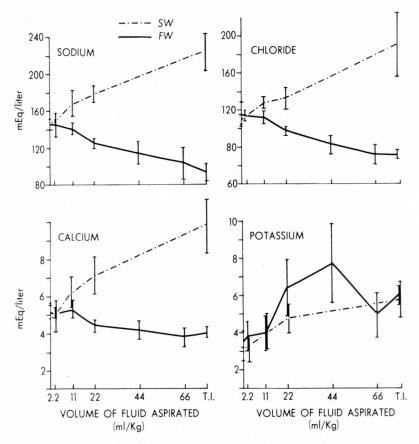

Figure 10. Serum electrolyte concentrations of arterial blood are plotted three minutes after aspiration of varying quantities of fresh water (FW) and sea water (SW). The volume of fluid aspirated ranged from 2.2 ml/kg to total immersion (TI). The line graph represents the mean of each group and the standard deviation is also indicated. (Modified with permission from *Anesthesiology, 27*:662-672, 1966; *Ann Intern Med, 67*:68-80, 1967, and *Die Therapiewoche, 43*:1-7, 1968.)

near-drowning and drowning[4] are more likely to be the main factors in causing hyperkalemia.[2]

In dogs that survived near-drowning without therapy, the changes in serum sodium, chloride, potassium, and calcium observed immediately after aspiration returned to normal within one to two hours.[2,5,6] However, when very large quantities of fluid were aspirated, e.g. under conditions of total immersion, profound changes in serum electrolytes occurred.[2,7-9]

Most of the experimental data on serum electrolyte changes after drowning and near-drowning have been collected in dogs. Although sodium and potassium concentrations in serum are similar in man and dog, the concentrations of these two electrolytes in erythrocytes are reversed[3] (man: K $= 136$ mEq/liter, Na $= 19$ mEq/liter; dog: K $= 10$ mEq/liter, Na $= 135$ mEq/liter). Since hemolysis occurs after fresh water aspiration, releasing both ions into the plasma, direct comparison of data collected in these two species must be questioned. The rabbit, on the other hand, has erythrocytes with concentrations of potassium and sodium similar to those in humans[3] (K $= 142$ mEq/liter, Na $= 22$ mEq/liter). Rabbits that aspirated 22 ml of fresh water per kilogram body weight showed a fall in serum concentration of less than 20 mEq/ liter while sodium decreased at least 40 mEq/liter after aspiration of 44 ml/kg. The potassium concentration was also related to the quantity of water aspirated,[10] remaining essentially unchanged after aspiration of 22 ml/kg, but increasing after aspiration of 44 ml/kg.

When these changes in sodium observed in the rabbit were compared with those found in dogs,[2,5] there was no significant difference between the two species after aspiration of 22 ml/kg of distilled water. When 44 ml/kg were aspirated, the decrease in serum sodium was greater in the rabbit than in the dog; however, no significant differences were seen between changes in the two species in serum potassium and chloride.[10] The difference between sodium levels in the rabbit and dog after aspirating 44 ml/kg can be attributed to the release of sodium from hemolyzed erythrocytes in the dog. One might expect the potassium level to be higher in the rabbit for similar reasons; however, comparable increases were seen in both species. This could be because the release of potassium secondary to acute severe hypoxia in both species is of far greater magnitude than the potassium released by hemolysis of rabbit red cells. These data suggest that it is reasonable to compare serum electrolyte changes in rabbits, dogs, and man following aspiration of 22 ml of fresh water per kilogram of body weight. When levels of serum sodium in the dog after aspiration of 44 ml/kg are used for comparison with rabbits (and presumably humans), the volume of water aspirated in the latter two species will be overestimated.

In 1963, Fuller[11,12] reported that abnormal serum electrolyte concentrations were not a clinical problem in his patients suffering from near-drowning. This author's experience confirms Fuller's observations. In 16 victims of fresh water near-drowning who had blood samples drawn in the emergency room before therapy was started, severe changes in serum electrolyte concentrations were not found[12,13] (Table VII).

TABLE VII

SERUM ELECTROLYTE CONCENTRATIONS OF HUMAN VICTIMS
OF FRESH WATER NEAR-DROWNING

	Sodium (mEq/liter)			Chloride (mEq/liter)			Potassium (mEq/liter)		
	# pts	mean	range	# pts	mean	range	# pts	mean	range
Fuller[12]	6	138	130-146	9	105	95-116	5	4.8	3.4-6.2
Modell*	16	137	126-146	16	98	88-106	16	4.3	3.0-6.3
Totals	22	137	126-146	25	101	88-116	21	4.4	3.0-6.3

*Six of these patients have been reported previously.[13]

SEA WATER

Following sea water aspiration, the changes in serum electrolyte concentrations are directly proportional to the volume of water aspirated. Although significant changes in serum chloride, sodium, potassium, and calcium did not occur after aspiration of 2.2 ml of sea water per kilogram body weight, there was a significant increase in all four electrolytes when dogs aspirated 11 ml/kg or more. The changes in electrolyte concentrations seen in Figure 10 three minutes after aspiration are plotted as a function of the quantity of water aspirated.[14] The profound changes in sodium and chloride concentrations found in this study after total immersion are comparable to the earlier results reported by Swann.[7-9] Sea water also contains a high concentration of magnesium. In the few studies in dogs where serum magnesium levels were quantitated, a significant increase was seen after total immersion.[8]

As was found in the experimental studies of fresh water aspiration, the electrolyte changes found after sea water aspiration spontaneously reverted to normal in dogs that survived without therapy. The serum calcium and potassium returned to normal within an hour in survivors, but the sodium and, particularly, the chloride concentrations remained elevated for a few hours in some animals.[14]

A composite series[12,13,15-17] of the serum sodium, chloride, and potassium concentrations seen in human victims of near-drowning in sea water is shown in Table VIII. The range of values in the

TABLE VIII

SERUM ELECTROLYTE CONCENTRATIONS IN HUMAN VICTIMS
OF SEA WATER NEAR-DROWNING

	Sodium (mEq/liter)			*Chloride (mEq/liter)*			*Potassium (mEq/liter)*		
	# pts	*mean*	*range*	*# pts*	*mean*	*range*	*# pts*	*mean*	*range*
Fuller[12]	5	150	142-158	7	112	96-127	5	4.4	3.5-4.9
Cahill[15]	6	145	136-151	7	108	100-115	6	4.3	3.5-5.4
Modell*	12	149	137-160	12	113	100-120	12	4.0	3.2-4.4
Misc.[16,17]	3	142	132-150	2	111	101-111	2	4.2	3.8-4.6
Totals	26	147	132-160	28	111	96-127	25	4.2	3.2-5.4

*Six of these patients have been reported previously.[13]

table shows that some patients had a significant increase in sodium or chloride concentration on admission to the hospital. Potassium concentrations were frequently lower than expected. In no case, however, were these values sufficiently abnormal to be considered life-threatening. Similar observations have been made by Hasan *et al.*[18] in their series of 32 victims of near-drowning in sea water. Therefore, serum electrolyte changes have not yet presented problems requiring correction in the emergency treatment of the near-drowning victim.

SIGNIFICANCE OF ELECTROLYTE CHANGES

It appears from the above observations of human near-drowning victims that the changes in serum electrolyte concentrations after both fresh and sea water near-drowning do not play a major role in determining patient survival. Yet, when large quantities of fluid are aspirated, e.g. under conditions of total immersion, there is no question that profound electrolyte changes can occur.

In a recent study, sera obtained from the left ventricle of 118 drowning victims were analyzed for concentration of serum electrolytes. The values found were then compared to a group of control patients, i.e. patients who died acutely from causes other than drowning. The mean values and standard deviations for serum chloride, sodium, and potassium are listed in Table IX. In order

TABLE IX

MEANS AND STANDARD DEVIATIONS OF SERUM ELECTROLYTE CONCENTRATIONS AND
SPECIFIC GRAVITY OF SAMPLES OBTAINED FROM THE LEFT VENTRICLE OF
PATIENTS WHO DIED OF FRESH WATER DROWNING, SEA WATER
DROWNING, OR OTHER CAUSES (CONTROLS)

	Fresh Water Victims 74 Patients	*FW vs. Control P Value*	*Controls* 24 Patients	*Control vs. SW P Value*	*Sea Water Victims* 44 Patients	*FW vs. SW P Value*
Cl mEq/liter	89 ± 11.4	*	93 ± 8.7	<0.001	120 ± 16.8	<0.001
Na mEq/liter	128 ± 11.5	<0.01	135 ± 9.9	<0.001	150 ± 12.5	<0.001
K mEq/liter	18.2 ± 7.4	*	18.6 ± 9.1	*	16.1 ± 6.6	*
Specific gravity	1.0280 ± 0.0040	<0.01	1.0309 ± 0.0046	*	1.0307 ± 0.0037	<0.01

*No significant difference between groups P > 0.10.
Modified with permission from *Anesthesiology, 30*:414-420, 1969.

to correlate these data with those from animal experiments, a frequency distribution of serum chloride and sodium concentrations has been listed in Table X. While the mean concentration of serum sodium in the left ventricle was significantly less in the victims of

TABLE X

FREQUENCY DISTRIBUTION OF SERUM SODIUM AND CHLORIDE CONCENTRATIONS OF
BLOOD DRAWN FROM THE LEFT VENTRICLE OF HUMAN
DROWNING VICTIMS AND NON-DROWNING CONTROLS

	Serum Chloride (mEq/liter)				*Serum Sodium (mEq/liter)*			
#pts	≤79	80-125	126-135	≥136	≤119	120-160	161-170	≥170
Controls	24	1	23	0	0	1	23	0	0
Sea water victims	44	0	26	11	7	0	39	4	1
Fresh water victims	74	10	63	1	0	12	61	1	0

Modified with permission from *Anesthesiology, 30*:414-420, 1969.

fresh water drowning than in the control patients, mean chloride and potassium concentrations in the two groups were not different. In only ten of 74 victims of fresh water drowning[19] (14%) was the concentration of serum chloride in the left ventricle less than 80 mEq/liter and in only 12 (16%) was the serum sodium less than 120 mEq/liter. Dogs that aspirated 22 ml/kg or less of fresh water had changes in sodium and chloride concentrations of less than 20 mEq/liter three minutes after aspiration, and aspiration of 44 ml/kg produced values more than 20 mEq/liter below normal.[2] If the animal data can be extrapolated to humans, approximately 85 percent of these human fresh water drowning victims aspirated 22 ml/kg of fluid or less. Animals that aspirated this quantity of fluid had electrolyte changes which spontaneously returned to normal.[2,5] Therefore, the majority of these patients probably did not die acutely of electrolyte imbalance and/or ventricular fibrillation[19] (see Chap. VIII).

Similarly, the results seen in the 44 victims of sea water drowning reported by us[19] can be compared to animal studies. When the frequency distribution of the serum chloride samples was analyzed, 59 percent of the patients had chloride values within 20 mEq/liter of normal. An additional 25 percent had values between 21 and 30 mEq/liter above normal. These data can be compared to animal data where three minutes after aspiration of 11 ml/kg of sea water the average increase in serum chloride concentration was less than 20 mEq/liter. When 22 ml/kg of sea water was aspirated,[14] the mean increase was more than 20 but less than 30 mEq/liter. From these data, it might be inferred that 59 percent of sea water drowning victims aspirated 11 ml/kg or less of sea water, that 25 percent aspirated between 11 and 22 ml/kg, and that only 16 percent aspirated more than 22 ml/kg. These data closely resemble the findings in the fresh water drowning victims,[19] where only 14 percent were estimated to have aspirated more than 22 ml/kg.

The results of these studies suggest that human near-drowning victims, and the majority of human drowning victims, die of causes other than acute electrolyte changes. If changes do occur, they likely will not be severe and will revert to normal without specific therapy. These results cast considerable doubt on the value or advisability of infusing distilled water intravenously into all sea water drowning victims, or hypertonic saline into all fresh water drowning victims as has been recommended by some authors.[20] The use of these solutions likely can cause more severe disturbances in serum electrolytes than those caused by the near-drowning episode itself. Furthermore, the time lost and diversion from treatment of the more important blood gas and acid-base changes may be crucial in determining whether or not the patient will survive.

The data presented above should not be interpreted to imply that significant changes in electrolytes which may compromise survival never occur during the drowning episode. Kylstra,[21] in his classic experiment of subjecting mice to total immersion in fresh water, sea water, and normal saline solution under 8 atmospheres of oxygen, has clearly shown that the survival times are different in these three fluids. The mice he studied in fresh water lived from 5.7 to 6.1 minutes. Those submerged in sea water lived from 11.0 to 11.5 minutes, and those in normal saline solution from 22 to 40 minutes. It is likely that these differences in survival time were related to changes in blood volume and electrolyte concentrations, which resulted from breathing the hypo- and hypertonic fluids.

Summary

The magnitude and direction of the changes in concentration of serum electrolytes which occur following near-drowning and drowning are dependent upon both the tonicity and the volume of water aspirated. The available data suggest that approximately 85 percent of humans who die of drowning, and presumably most all who survive, aspirated less than 22 ml/kg of water. This quantity of aspirated fluid does not, of itself, produce life-threatening changes in serum electrolyte concentrations. Therefore, correction of electrolyte disturbances is of secondary rather than primary importance in the treatment of most human victims of near-drowning.

REFERENCES

1. Revenstorf: Über den Wert der Kryoskopie zur Diagnose des Todes durch Ertrinken. *München Med Wschr, 49*:1880, 1902.
2. Modell, J. H., and Moya, F.: Effects of volume of aspirated fluid during chlorinated fresh water drowning. *Anesthesiology, 27*:662-672, 1966.
3. Bernstein, R. E.: Potassium and sodium balance in mammalian red cells. *Science, 120*:459-460, 1954.

4. Butt, M. P.; Jalowayski, A.; Modell, J. H., and Giammona, S. T.: Pulmonary function after resuscitation from near-drowning. *Anesthesiology, 32*:275-277, 1970.
5. Modell, J. H.; Gaub, M.; Moya, F.; Vestal, B., and Swarz, H.: Physiologic effects of near drowning with chlorinated fresh water, distilled water and isotonic saline. *Anesthesiology, 27*:33-41, 1966.
6. Farthmann, E. H., and Davidson, A. I. G.: Fresh water drowning at lowered body temperature; an experimental study. *Amer J Surg, 109*: 410-415, 1965.
7. Fainer, D. C.; Martin, C. G., and Ivy, A. C.: Resuscitation of dogs from fresh water drowning. *J Appl Physiol, 3*:417-426, 1951.
8. Swann, H. G., and Spafford, N. R.: Body salt and water changes during fresh and sea water drowning. *Texas Rep Biol Med, 9*:356-382, 1951.
9. Swann, H. G.; Brucer, M.; Moore, C., and Vezien, B. L.: Fresh water and sea water drowning: A study of the terminal cardiac and biochemical events. *Texas Rep Biol Med, 5*:423-437, 1947.
10. Modell, J. H.; Weibley, T. C.; Ruiz, B. C., and Newby, E. J.: Serum electrolyte concentrations after fresh-water aspiration: a comparison of species. *Anesthesiology, 30*:421-425, 1969.
11. Fuller, R. H.: The 1962 Wellcome prize essay. Drowning and the postimmersion syndrome. A clinicopathologic study. *Milit Med. 128*:22-36, 1963.
12. Fuller, R. H.: The clinical pathology of human near-drowning. *Proc Roy Soc Med, 56*:33-38, 1963.
13. Modell, J. H.; Davis, J. H.; Giammona, S. T.; Moya, F., and Mann, J. B.: Blood gas and electrolyte changes in human near-drowning victims. *JAMA, 203*:337-343, 1968.
14. Modell, J. H.; Moya, F.; Newby, E. J.; Ruiz, B. C., and Showers, A. V.: The effects of fluid volume in seawater drowning. *Ann Intern Med, 67*:68-80, 1967.
15. Cahill, J. H.: Drowning; the problem of nonfatal submersion and the unconscious patient. *Surg Clin N Amer, 48*:423-430, 1968.
16. Fainer, D. C.: Near drowning in sea water and fresh water. *Ann Intern Med, 59*:537-541, 1963.
17. Warden, J. C.: Respiratory insufficiency following near-drowning in sea water. *JAMA, 201*:887-890, 1967.
18. Hasan, S.; Avery, W. G.; Fabian, C., and Sackner, M. A.: Near drowning in humans. A report of 36 patients. *Chest, 59*:191-197, 1971.
19. Modell, J. H., and Davis, J. H.: Electrolyte changes in human drowning victims. *Anesthesiology, 30*:414-420, 1969.
20. Shaw, C. C.: "Man Overboard." *Med Tech Bull, 7*:193-198, 1956.
21. Kylstra, J. A.: Drowning: The rôle of salts in the drowning fluid; a preliminary report on observations in mice. *Acta Physiol Pharmacol Neerl, 10*:327-334, 1961.

Chapter VII

HEMOGLOBIN, HEMATOCRIT, HEMOLYSIS, AND PLATELETS

T HE HEMOGLOBIN AND HEMATOCRIT concentrations measured in humans after near-drowning are usually normal, suggesting that most near-drowning victims do not aspirate large quantities of fluid. However, when hypo- and hypertonic fluids come in contact with red blood cells, changes in cell size occur. This can lead to difficulties in interpretation of the values.

EXPERIMENTAL FRESH WATER DROWNING AND NEAR-DROWNING

Hemoglobin

In 1949, Swann and Brucer[1] reported that whole blood hemoglobin fell precipitously in dogs between the third and fifth minute after drowning by total immersion in fresh water.[1,2] Yet, Farthmann and Davidson[3] and Modell *et al.*[4,5] did not find a significant drop in hemoglobin concentration after fresh water aspiration. One significant difference between Swann's studies[1,2] and those of Farthmann and Davidson[3] and of Modell *et al.*[4,5] was that Swann's dogs were not anesthetized. Those in the latter studies were under barbiturate anesthesia. Hahn *et al.*[6] pointed out that up to 30 percent of the dog's red blood cell volume was pooled in the spleen during barbiturate anesthesia. When lightly anesthetized animals were subjected to aspiration, the spleen may have contracted and an increase in circulating red blood cells resulted. Normal anesthetized dogs show an increase in hemoglobin concentration three minutes after aspiration of 22 ml/kg of fresh water. However, a slight decrease in hemoglobin results if the animals have had a splenectomy prior to aspiration[5] (Fig. 11). Hemoglobin changes after drowning and near-drowning have also been studied in other species. The hemoglobin concentration remained unchanged in the rabbit after aspiration of 22 ml/kg of fresh water. Yet, after drowning in 44 ml/kg, a significant fall in hemoglobin concentration occurred.[7] Unlike changes in blood volume and serum electrolyte concentrations, the hemoglobin concentration after near-drowning in fresh water cannot be directly correlated with the volume of water aspirated.[5]

Another problem in evaluating the changes in hemoglobin im-

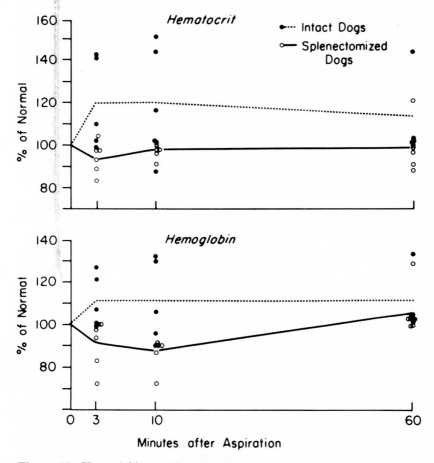

Figure 11. Hemoglobin and hematocrit concentrations after aspiration of 22 ml/kg of fresh water are compared between intact dogs and dogs that have had a prior splenectomy. All values are reported as percent of pre-aspiration level. The values for individual animals are plotted as well as the mean for each group.

mediately after fresh water aspiration is related to the method of measurement. Most commonly, the cyanmethemoglobin method is used. The red blood cells are hemolyzed and the hemoglobin concentration is read as a color reaction in a spectrophotometer. During drowning, if significant quantities of fresh water are aspirated, hemolysis occurs, releasing hemoglobin into the plasma. What is read with colorimetric tests is then the total hemoglobin concentration, rather than the hemoglobin within red blood cells. Unless the plasma hemoglobin concentration is measured independently and subtracted, this limits the clinical interpretation and application of such determinations immediately after fresh water aspiration.

Hematocrit

Hematocrit determinations have not been reported in experimental animals that were drowned while they were awake. Under barbiturate anesthesia, the hematocrit increased after aspiration of fresh water in dogs[3,5] (Fig. 12). Splenectomy did not have as

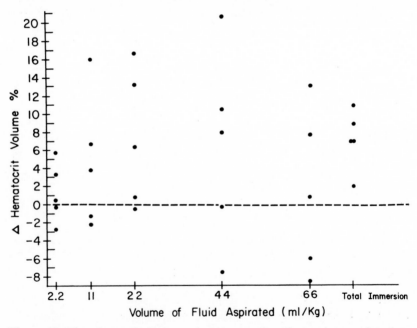

Figure 12. The change in hematocrit concentration three minutes after dogs aspirated fresh water is plotted against the volume of fluid aspirated (Reprinted with permission from *Anesthesiology, 27*:662-672, 1966).

marked an effect on hematocrit values seen after aspiration as it did on hemoglobin concentration (Fig. 11). Thus, the release of red cells from the spleen may account for part of the rise in hematocrit, but it does not fully explain its magnitude.

Farthmann and Davidson[3] attributed the increase in hematocrit found in their animals to the loss of plasma as pulmonary edema fluid. An additional factor has been shown to contribute to the increase in hematocrit, i.e. with the influx of hypotonic solution into the bloodstream, the red cells swell and assume a greater volume. The magnitude of change is limited by the capacity and fragility of the cells. If a significant number of cells increase in size, but not to the point of rupture, although some hemolysis may occur, the net result would be an increase in hematocrit. This effect can be demonstrated by the following, simple experiment.

Five milliliters of venous blood were drawn from each of five normal animals and diluted with distilled water to a total volume of 7.5 ml. Three minutes following the addition of the water, microcapillary tubes containing the diluted blood were prepared and the hematocrit was determined. The predicted and actual

TABLE XI

PREDICTED VS MEASURED HEMATOCRIT VALUES OF HEPARINIZED BLOOD THREE
MINUTES AFTER DILUTION TO 150 PERCENT OF NORMAL VOLUME
WITH DISTILLED WATER

Dog Number	Pre-dilution Hematocrit (vol%)	After Dilution Hematocrit		Measured Minus Predicted Hematocrit (vol%)
		Predicted (vol%)	Measured (vol%)	
1	26.2	17.5	23.5	6.0
2	22.5	15.0	20.0	5.0
3	35.5	26.7	31.5	5.2
4	22.0	14.7	19.5	4.8
5	31.5	21.0	28.3	7.3
Average	27.5	18.9	24.6	5.7

hematocrit values following dilution of the blood are seen in Table XI. If the red cell size remained constant and all relative changes were due to pure dilution, the average hematocrit would have dropped from 27.5 vol% to 18.9 vol%. This was not the case, however, as the average decline in hematocrit was only 2.0 vol%. The difference between the actual and predicted values, 5.7 vol%, may be attributed to an increase in the red cell size due to swelling from the hypotonic solution (Modell, J. H., and Zies, P., unpublished data). Therefore, the reliability of the hematocrit concentration as a guide for detecting hemodilution from aspiration of hypotonic fluid is limited.

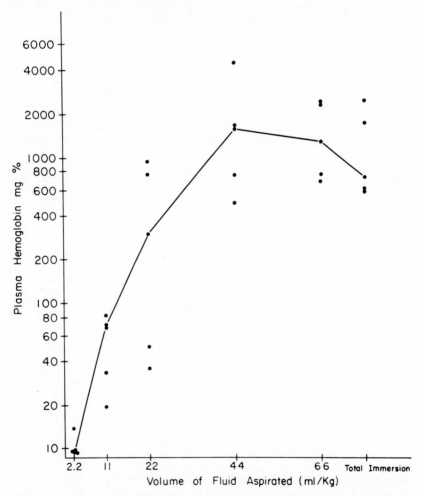

Figure 13. The plasma hemoglobin concentration determined three minutes after aspiration of fresh water is plotted against the volume of fluid aspirated (Reprinted with permission from *Anesthesiology, 27*:662-672, 1966).

Plasma Hemoglobin and Hemolysis

When small quantities of fresh water are aspirated, no significant hemolysis occurs. However, plasma hemoglobin concentration has been shown to increase proportionately as increasing volumes of fluid are aspirated by dogs[5] (Fig. 13). The plasma hemoglobin concentration reached a plateau when the volume of water aspirated was sufficient to produce ventricular fibrillation in 80 percent of the dogs tested.[5]

Since the volume of fluid aspirated has not been held constant by all investigators, considerable differences in plasma hemoglobin levels have been reported. Spitz and Blanke[8] reported the plasma hemoglobin concentration to be between 96 and 1,458 mg% within 30 seconds, and 185 to 3,000 mg% within 60 seconds of total immersion. Eleven of their 15 dogs had levels below 1,000 mg% at one minute. Farthmann and Davidson[3] reported the plasma hemoglobin concentration as having ranged between 100 and 4,800 mg% (mean 1,330 mg%) 15 minutes after near-drowning under hypothermia. The highest serum hemoglobin level reported by Swann[9] after total immersion in fresh water was 7,000 mg%.

Fainer, Martin and Ivy[10] found that six of seven untreated animals survived when the plasma hemoglobin level after fresh water aspiration was less than 500 mg%. Only one out of 29 survived if it was higher. Unfortunately, the amount of water aspirated in these experiments was not stated. In our own experiments,[5] the highest plasma hemoglobin level three minutes postaspiration, followed by long-term survival of the animals, was 477 mg%. Two additional animals with levels of 740 mg% initially survived the aspiration only to die within twenty-four hours.

EXPERIMENTAL SEA WATER DROWNING AND NEAR-DROWNING

Hemoglobin and hematocrit concentrations of dogs remained stable after aspiration of small quantities of sea water (2.2 ml/kg). As larger quantities were aspirated, however, significant increases in both hemoglobin[1,11,12] and hematocrit[11] were seen. This increase correlated with the volume of water aspirated during near-drowning,[11] but varied considerably after total immersion.[1,11,12] The change in hemoglobin and hematocrit concentrations observed after aspiration of sea water by dogs was subject to the same variation between anesthetized and unanesthetized animals as reported after fresh water drowning. After sea water drowning, there was also a decrease in mean corpuscular volume[11] which resulted in an over-estimation of the relative loss of plasma to cells. Hemolysis was not a prominent feature after sea water aspiration. Following near-drowning in sea water, the changes in hemoglobin and hematocrit were transient, and within hours, both returned to normal in the animals that survived.

HUMAN DROWNING AND NEAR-DROWNING

Since some hemolysis occurs postmortem regardless of the cause of death, hemoglobin and hematocrit concentrations in blood from drowning victims do not necessarily reflect premortem values. The hemoglobin and hematocrit values reported in patients soon after near-drowning in fresh water are shown in the composite Table XII.[13-18] It is particularly significant that only one patient of the 34 reported, an eleven-month-old child, had a hemoglobin concentration of less than 11.4 gm%. In many patients, the hemo-

TABLE XII

HEMOGLOBIN AND HEMATOCRIT CONCENTRATIONS
AFTER NEAR-DROWNING IN FRESH WATER

	Hemoglobin (gm%)		
	Number of Patients	*Range*	*Mean*
Fuller[13]	15	11.4-21.0	14.4
Modell[14]	6	12.0-14.0	13.0
Modell (unreported)	11	9.2-21.5	14.8
Miscellaneous[15,16]	2	14.5-16.3	15.4
Totals	34	9.2-21.5	14.2
	Hematocrit (vol%)		
	Number of Patients	*Range*	*Mean*
Fuller[13]	12	44-65	50
Modell[14]	6	36-44	40
Modell (unreported)	11	30-56	43
Cahill[17]	3	34-39	37
Miscellaneous[15,18]	2	48-51	50
Totals	34	30-65	44

globin and hematocrit values were higher than might be expected after aspiration of a hypotonic solution. This could be due to errors in measurement, as discussed above, to loss of plasma into the lung and other extravascular spaces, or to the fact that these patients aspirated small quantities of water. These observations suggest that hemoglobin and hematocrit concentrations are an unreliable guide on which to base therapy in the fresh water near-drowning victim.

Some patients demonstrate gross hemoglobinemia even though they have normal concentrations of hemoglobin and hematocrit.[13-15] In one series, plasma hemoglobin determinations were performed on all patients and values as high as 500 mg% were reported.[14] Fainer[18] reports a patient who survived near-drowning whose plasma hemoglobin level was 1,000 mg%. The use of exchange transfusions to treat massive hemolysis after near-drowning in fresh water has been advocated by some authors. Support for this approach comes from an experiment in dogs where the survival time was prolonged with partial exchange transfusions.[19] Also, there is one case reported in the literature where exchange transfusions were carried out in man.[20] In this patient, however, the serum hemoglobin level was only 177 mg%. Since this is lower than the levels in some survivors reported by other authors,[14,18] the patient may have survived because of, or in spite of, the exchange transfusions. It is likely that patients who aspirated quantities of fluid large enough to cause massive hemolysis are not recovered from the water alive. Thus, the value of exchange transfusion seems quite limited.

It is not unusual for normal hemoglobin and hematorcit concentrations to be found when the patient is admitted to the hospital, and yet, a significant fall in both is seen approximately twenty-four hours later.[14,15] This suggests that although hemodilution and hemolysis occur, limitations in the methods of determining hemoglobin and hematocrit concentrations prevent their detection until the hypotonic fluid and free hemoglobin have been removed from the blood. Since the hemoglobin concentration is the primary determinant of the oxygen carrying capacity of the blood, and near-drowning victims are prone to have difficulty in oxygenation, serial hemoglobin and hematocrit determinations should be done. If a significant fall in hemoglobin occurs, transfusion of whole blood must be considered.

The hemoglobin concentrations in 39 patients and the hematocrit concentrations in 52 patients after near-drowning in sea water are shown in Table XIII.[13,14,17,18,21] While a handful of patients showed

TABLE XIII

HEMOGLOBIN AND HEMATOCRIT CONCENTRATIONS
AFTER NEAR-DROWNING IN SEA WATER

	Hemoglobin (gm%)		
	Number of Patients	*Range*	*Mean*
Fuller[13]	26	12.3-19.8	14.7
Modell[14]	6	12.0-18.0	15.0
Modell (unreported)	4	12.0-15.0	13.5
Miscellaneous[18,21]	3	14.6-18.4	16.9
Totals	39	12.0-19.8	14.8
	Hematocrit (vol%)		
	Number of Patients	*Range*	*Mean*
Fuller[13]	27	36-55	45
Cahill[17]	12	31-50	39
Modell[14]	6	36-51	40
Modell (unreported)	4	36-42	40
Miscellaneous[18,21]	3	42-56	48
Totals	52	31-56	43

hemoglobin and hematocrit concentrations suggesting hemoconcentration, the majority of patients had normal values. The mean values from these patients are not different from those of the patients after fresh water near-drowning shown in Table XII.[13-18] Hasan *et al.* also failed to demonstrate abnormal hemoglobin and hematocrit values in 32 victims of sea water near-drowning.[22] These data suggest that large volumes of water are not aspirated by most patients who suffer a near-drowning episode. This would support the conclusion, based on electrolye changes, that 85 percent of all drowning victims aspirated less than 22 ml/kg of water (Chap. VI). Hemolysis is not a common occurrence after sea water aspiration, although one case of hemoglobinemia has been reported after aspiration of hypertonic fluid in the Great Salt Lake.[13]

PLATELETS

While no studies are available regarding specific clotting defects after near-drowning, masses of agglutinated platelets have been reported at autopsy in larger blood vessels, particularly those of the lung.[23] The relationship of these agglutinative platelet thrombi, apparently agonal, to the fact that clotting of blood postmortem usually is not seen after drowning, is speculative. Definitive studies are necessary before any conclusions are warranted regarding this matter.

Summary

Hemoglobin and hematocrit concentrations are usually normal in victims of both fresh and sea water near-drowning. This may be due to the fact that these patients do not aspirate large quantities of fluid. On the other hand, technical problems in measurement also limit interpretation of these values in the period immediately after near-drowning. While hemolysis does occur after aspiration of at least 11 ml/kg of fresh water, it seldom is of a magnitude which requires specific therapy in human near-drowning victims reported to date.

REFERENCES

1. Swann, H. G., and Brucer, M.: The cardiorespiratory and biochemical events during rapid anoxic death. VI. Fresh water and sea water drowning. *Texas Rep Biol Med, 7*:604-618, 1949.
2. Swann, H. G.; Brucer, M.; Moore, C., and Vezien, B. L.: Fresh water and sea water drowning: A study of the terminal cardiac and biochemical events. *Texas Rep Biol Med, 5*:423-437, 1947.
3. Farthmann, E. H., and Davidson, A. I. G.: Fresh water drowning at lowered body temperature; an experimental study. *Amer J Surg, 109*: 410-415, 1965.
4. Modell, J. H.; Gaub, M.; Moya, F.; Vestal, B., and Swarz, H.: Physiologic effects of near drowning with chlorinated fresh water, distilled water and isotonic saline. *Anesthesiology, 27*:33-41, 1966.
5. Modell, J. H., and Moya, F.: Effects of volume of aspirated fluid during chlorinated fresh water drowning. *Anesthesiology, 27*:662-672, 1966.
6. Hahn, P. F.; Bale, W. F., and Bonner, Jr., J. F.: Removal of red cells from active circulation by sodium pentobarbital. *Amer J Physiol, 138*:415-420, 1943.
7. Modell, J. H.; Weibley, T. C.; Ruiz, B. C., and Newby, E. J.: Serum electrolyte concentrations after fresh-water aspiration; a comparison

of species. *Anesthesiology, 30*:421-425, 1969.

8. Spitz, W. U., and Blanke, R. V.: Mechanism of death in fresh-water drowning. I. An experimental approach to the problem. *Arch Path (Chicago), 71*:661-668, 1961.

9. Swann, H. G.: Studies in Resuscitation. Mem. Rep. Aero M. Lab. (MCREXD-696-79J). U. S. Air Force (no. 6006), pp. 1-74, October, 1950.

10. Fainer, D. C.; Martin, C. G., and Ivy, A. C.: Resuscitation of dogs from fresh water drowning. *J Appl Physiol, 3*:417-426, 1951.

11. Modell, J. H.; Moya, F.; Newby, E. J.; Ruiz, B. C., and Showers, A. V.: The effects of fluid volume in seawater drowning. *Ann Intern Med, 67*:68-80, 1967.

12. Swann, H. G., and Spafford, N. R.: Body salt and water changes during fresh and sea water drowning. *Texas Rep Biol Med, 9*:356-382, 1951.

13. Fuller, R. H.: The clinical pathology of human near-drowning. *Proc Roy Soc Med, 56*:33-38, 1963.

14. Modell, J. H.; Davis, J. H.; Giammona, S. T.; Moya, F., and Mann, J. B.: Blood gas and electrolyte changes in human near-drowning victims. *JAMA, 203*:337-343, 1968.

15. Munroe, W. D.: Hemoglobinuria from near-drowning. *J Pediat, 64*:57-62, 1964.

16. Haddy, T. B., and Disenhouse, R. B.: Acute pulmonary edema due to near-drowning in fresh water. *J Pediat, 44*:565-569, 1954.

17. Cahill, J. M.: Drowning: the problem of nonfatal submersion and the unconscious patient. *Surg Clin N Amer, 48*:423-430, 1968.

18. Fainer, D. C.: Near drowning in sea water and fresh water. *Ann Intern Med, 59*:537-541, 1963.

19. Spitz, W. U.: Recovery from drowning. *Brit Med J, 5346*:1678, 1963.

20. Kvittingen, T. D., and Naess, A.: Recovery from drowning in fresh water. *Brit Med J, 5341*:1315-1317, 1963.

21. Warden, J. C.: Respiratory insufficiency following near-drowning in sea water. *JAMA, 201*:887-890, 1967.

22. Hasan, S.; Avery, W. G.; Fabian, C., and Sackner, M. A.: Near drowning in humans. A report of 36 patients. *Chest, 59*:191-197, 1971.

23. Fuller, R. H.: The 1962 Wellcome prize essay. Drowning and the postimmersion syndrome. A clinicopathologic study. *Milit Med, 128*:22-36, 1963.

Chapter VIII

CARDIOVASCULAR SYSTEM

IN DESCRIBING THE CAUSE OF DEATH during drowning, many authors have emphasized the changes which occur in cardiovascular function.[1-4] Most human near-drowning victims, however, show remarkable stability of the cardiovascular system.[5,6] Recent experimental evidence suggests that changes in cardiovascular function during near-drowning and drowning are predominantly secondary to changes in arterial oxygen tension and acid-base balance.[4,5,7-9] Changes in blood volume and serum electrolyte concentrations obviously contribute to these changes, but apparently only to a limited degree as pointed out in Chapters III through VII. Significant blood volume and serum electrolyte changes are seen only when large volumes of water have been aspirated.

HEART

The most common finding in dogs immediately after aspiration of either fresh water[9-15] or sea water[7,12,14] was a bradycardia. If the animal survived the immediate postaspiration period, the heart rate increased and a tachycardia frequently occurred. Similar alterations in heart rate have been reported in human victims of near-drowning.[16,17] While electrocardiographic changes in experimental studies were usually limited to transient changes in heart rate after aspiration of 2.2 ml/kg of either fresh or sea water,[7,9] aspiration of larger quantities of water caused a wide variety of electrocardiographic abnormalities. A decrease in the amplitude of the P wave,[11,18] a disappearance of the P wave, a widened PR interval,[11,18] complete A-V dissociation[11,13,15] and depression of the ST segment[18] all have been reported after aspiration of either fresh or sea water. When fresh water was aspirated, widening of the QRS complex[18] with frequent premature ventricular contractions[10,15] and an increase in amplitude of the T wave[9-11] have also been observed in some instances. When at least 44 ml/kg

61

of fresh water was aspirated, ventricular fibrillation occurred in 80 percent of dogs studied.[9] Swann and Brucer have described the electrocardiographic changes which preceded death in dogs after total immersion in fresh water as a dissociation of auricular and ventricular complexes with concomitant bradycardia, followed by auricular fibrillation and an increase in the amplitude of the T wave. The T wave then merged with the ST segment, the amplitude of the R wave increased until the QT complex became monophasic, and ventricular fibillation occurred. After total immersion in sea water, their dogs showed a lengthening of the PR interval with dissociation of the auricular-ventricular complexes, ST segment elevation, inverted T waves, and a decrease in amplitude of the R wave.[11] Ventricular fibrillation during total immersion of dogs in sea water has been reported only once.[19]

A correlation of the changes in serum sodium and chloride in blood taken from the left ventricle of human drowning victims with those seen in experimental animals suggests that only 15 percent of the humans who drowned in fresh water aspirated sufficient quantities of water to produce ventricular fibrillation.[20,21] Ventricular fibrillation in human victims of drowning has been documented only on two occasions: one after aspiration of sea water[22] and the other after fresh water aspiration.[23] It is likely that humans who aspirate sufficient fluid to produce ventricular fibrillation are not retrieved from the water alive since, in dogs, fibrillation occurs within two to seven minutes of immersion.[9,24]

Since ventricular fibrillation, secondary to fresh water drowning, was first described in dogs by Banting *et al.*[25] in 1938, there has been considerable speculation as to its etiology. It has been suggested that ventricular fibrillation may be due to an increase in serum potassium concentration secondary to hemolysis, a decrease in serum calcium or sodium concentration due to hemodilution, or a combination of these.[1,4,26] Swann[26] found that parenteral administration of calcium did not prevent ventricular fibrillation during total immersion in fresh water. When sodium was injected, however, fibrillation did not occur even though the electrocardiogram showed the merged QRST complex which is so characterstic of approaching ventricular fibrillation. With the injection of sodium, the pattern of complexes rapidly reverted to a separation of the QRS and T waves; however, the ST segment remained elevated due to hypoxia. The same investigator[1,26] also demonstrated, through intravenous injection of large volumes of water in dogs, that fibrillation could not be produced solely by lowering the serum sodium. In addition to the hyponatremia, anoxia had to be present for fibrillation to occur. If, in the face of hypoxia, potassium increased but serum sodium was maintained at reasonably normal levels, ventricular fibrillation did not occur. From these studies, Swann concluded that the combination of acute profound hyponatremia and anoxia was responsible for the ventricular fibrillation seen after aspiration of large volumes of fresh water.[1]

Although an intravenous injection of sodium interrupted the progression of EKG changes leading toward ventricular fibrillation, once fibrillation occurred, injection of sodium chloride solution did not reverse the fibrillation.[1] Redding and his colleagues[2] have shown that ventricular fibrillation after fresh water aspiration can be terminated in dogs when intermittent positive pressure ventilation with 100% oxygen and closed chest cardiac massage are followed by electrical defibrillation.

Spitz and Blanke[27] reported that death from ventricular fibrillation in dogs was not a constant finding after aspiration of fresh water. They observed the electrocardiogram in eight dogs and only two demonstrated ventricular fibrillation. They concluded that the mechanism of death in those animals not developing ventricular fibrillation was the failure of an overloaded and hypoxic myocardium.

The fact that only one case of ventricular fibrillation in humans after fresh water drowning has been referred to in the literature raises the question of whether or not ventricular fibrillation might be a species variable phenomenon. By studying animals of various species, Gordon, Raymon, and Ivy[28] observed that ventricular fibrillation follows total immersion in fresh water in the horse, cow, sheep, goat, pig, and dog, but not in the white rat or guinea pig. In the cat, monkey, and rabbit, these authors reported that ventricular fibrillation occurred, but that it spontaneously reversed. Modell *et al.*, on the other hand, have shown that ventricular fibrillation with death can occur in the rabbit.[21] In view of our current knowledge, it seems likely that humans can die of ventricular fibrillation after fresh water aspiration. The reason it is not seen more often is that human victims of near-drowning, and 85 percent of those who die in the water, do not aspirate more than 22 ml of water per kilogram body weight. Since 44 ml/kg is the critical volume for production of ventricular fibrillation in dogs, it is likely that fibrillation occurs in less than 15 percent of human drowning victims. These 15 percent are not resuscitated and, therefore electrocardiographic monitoring is not obtained. This would explain why ventricular fibrillation in human drowning victims is not reported more frequently. In short, while ventricular fibrillation may be the immedate cause of death in a limited number of human victims of drowning, it is not a problem in the treatment of most patients who near-drown.

ARTERIAL BLOOD PRESSURE

Arterial blood pressure in human near-drowning victims varies considerably. For example, Fainer[16] reports that the blood pressure was not obtainable by usual manometric techniques in a victim of fresh water near-drowning. On the other hand, patients have been reported to be normotensive[29] and hypertensive[17,29-31] after a near-drowning episode. Much of this variability may be related to the time at which the blood pressure is taken relative to the near-drowning episode and to the adequacy of oxygenation since hypoxia affects adrenal activity, vessel tone, and myocardial function.

When blood pressure changes were observed under controlled experimental conditions in animals, only minor changes were seen after aspiration of 2.2 ml of water per kilogram body weight. There was a slight increase in systolic blood pressure which coincided with hyperventilation for approximately 15 minutes after aspiration. When as much as 11 ml/kg of fresh water was aspirated, there was a transient fall in arterial blood pressure of at least 30 torr, followed by an increase above normal which lasted up to one hour. When 44 ml/kg or more was aspirated, the initial response was similar.[9,10,13,27] The blood pressure then returned to normal over the next hour in the animals that survived, fell precipitously in those that died of ventricular fibrillation, or underwent a gradual but progressive fall in the animals that died without fibrillation.[9,10,27,32]

Following aspiration of at least 11 ml/kg of sea water, there usually was an immediate decrease in arterial pressure coinciding with a period of bradycardia.[7] This was followed by a return to preaspiration systolic levels or even hypertension.[7,26] In animals that died after aspiration of sea water, a gradual decline in arterial blood pressure occurred over a period of minutes. Swann[26] correlated the degree of hypotension with resuscitability in dogs and has reported that once the systolic blood pressure dropped below 100 torr, dogs could not be resuscitated from sea water aspiration. In Modell's studies, almost all animals that aspirated at least 22 ml/kg of sea water showed a fall in systolic blood pressure to below 100 torr within 30 seconds of aspiration. The blood pressure spontaneously rose above this figure only to begin a progressive decline, which terminated with the death of the animals.[7] If fluid had been drained from the lungs and active resuscitative measures had been applied early to these animals, it is possible that some may have survived.

The changes in arterial blood pressure may have a complex etiology since the blood pressure is the net result of a variety of factors: vascular tone, an increase or decrease in circulating catecholamines, peripheral vasoconstriction from immersion in cold fluid, the levels of CO_2 and O_2 tensions in arterial blood, changes in circulating blood volume due to aspiration of hypo- or hypertonic fluid, or loss of intravascular fluid because of changes in capillary permeability. Cardiac output will vary with many of these factors, as well as with changes in electrolyte concentrations. A changing cardiac output, in turn, will also affect the arterial blood pressure. It is important, therefore, to focus attention not so much on the absolute readings of arterial pressure but, rather, on the correction of the etiological factors involved.

CENTRAL VENOUS PRESSURE

Immediately after aspiration of small quantities of fresh or sea water, dogs demonstrate an increase in central venous pressure which coincides with periods of hyperventilation. Then, the central venous pressure rapidly returns to normal in all cases.[7,9] After aspiration of large quantities of fresh water, the rise in central venous pressure persists. In animals that die shortly after aspiration, it may never return to normal levels.[9,12,14,15,27] However, if the animal survives, there is a gradual return to a normal central venous pressure over a period of approximately one hour.[9,10] Following aspiration of large quantities of sea water, there is also an initial increase in central venous pressure.[7,12,14] This increase is transient, however, and the central venous pressure rapidly falls toward zero both in animals that survive and in those that die during total immersion.[12] This likely reflects the acute decrease in blood volume that occurs when plasma is lost into the lungs.

Summary

The nature and magnitude of changes in cardiovascular function after near-drowning and drowning vary both with the type and volume of fluid aspirated. They undoubtedly are most frequently secondary to hypoxia. When large volumes of water are aspirated, however, changes in blood volume and serum electrolyte concentrations may also influence cardiovascular function. Although death from ventricular fibrillation after fresh water aspiration has been stressed in the past, recent evidence indicates that it occurs infrequently in human drowning victims.

REFERENCES

1. Swann, H. G.: Editorial: Mechanism of circulatory failure in fresh and sea water drowning. *Circulat Res, 4*:241-244, 1956.
2. Redding, J. S., and Cozine, R. A.: Restoration of circulation after fresh water drowning. *J Appl Physiol, 16*:1071-1074, 1961.
3. Crosfill, J. W. L.: Drowning. *Proc Roy Soc Med, 49*:1051-1058, 1956.
4. Noble, C. S., and Sharpe, N.: Drowning; its mechanism and treatment. *Canad Med Ass J, 89*:402-405, 1963.
5. Modell, J. H.; Davis, J. H.; Giammona, S. T.; Moya, F., and Mann, J. B.: Blood gas and electrolyte changes in human near-drowning victims. *JAMA, 203*:337-343, 1968.
6. Hasan, S.; Avery, W. G.; Fabian, C., and Sackner, M. A.: Near drowning in humans. A report of 36 patients. *Chest, 59*:191-197, 1971.
7. Modell, J. H.; Moya, F.; Newby, E. J.; Ruiz, B. C., and Showers, A. V.: The effects of fluid volume in seawater drowning. *Ann Intern Med, 67*:68-80, 1967.
8. Modell, J. H.; Moya, F.; Williams, H. D., and Weibley, T. C.: Changes in blood gases and A-aDO$_2$ during near-drowning. *Anesthesiology, 29*:456-465, 1968.
9. Modell, J. H., and Moya, F.: Effects of volume of aspirated fluid during chlorinated fresh water drowning. *Anestehsiology, 27*:662-672, 1966.

10. Modell, J. H.; Gaub, M.; Moya, F.; Vestal, B., and Swarz, H.: Physiologic effects of near drowning with chlorinated fresh water, distilled water and isotonic saline. *Anesthesiology, 27*:33-41, 1966.
11. Swann, H. G., and Brucer, M.: The cardiorespiratory and biochemical events during rapid anoxic death. VI. Fresh water and sea water drowning. *Texas Rep Biol Med, 7*:604-618, 1949.
12. Swann, H. G.; Brucer, M.; Moore, C., and Vezien, B. L.: Fresh water and sea water drowning: A study of the terminal cardiac and biochemical events. *Texas Rep Biol Med, 5*:423-437, 1947.
13. Lougheed, D. W.; Janes, J. M., and Hall, G. E.: Physiological studies in experimental asphyxia and drowning. *Canad Med Ass J, 40*:423-428, 1939.
14. Redding, J.; Voigt, G. C., and Safar, P.: Drowning treated with intermittent positive pressure breathing. *J Appl Physiol, 15*:849-854, 1960.
15. Farthmann, E. H., and Davidson, A. I. G.: Fresh water drowning at lowered body temperature; an experimental study. *Amer J Surg, 109*:410-415, 1965.
16. Fainer, D. C.: Near drowning in sea water and fresh water. *Ann Intern Med, 59*:537-541, 1963.
17. Rath, C. E.: Drowning hemoglobinuria. *Blood, 8*:1099-1104, 1953.
18. Trethewie, E. R.: Cardio-vascular effects in drowning. *Cardiologia (Basel), 33*:423-434, 1958.
19. Giammona, S. T., and Modell, J. H.: Drowning by total immersion. Effects on pulmonary surfactant of distilled water, isotonic saline and sea water. *Amer J Dis Child, 114*:612-616, 1967.
20. Modell, J. H., and Davis, J. H.: Electrolyte changes in human drowning victims. *Anesthesiology, 30*:414-420, 1969.
21. Modell, J. H.; Weibley, T.C.; Ruiz, B.C., and Newby, E. J.: Serum electrolyte concentrations after fresh-water aspiration: a comparison of species. *Anesthesiology, 30*:421-425, 1969.
22. Middleton, K. R.: Cardiac arrest induced by drowning: attempted resuscitation by external and internal cardiac massage. *Canad Med Ass J, 86*:374-375, 1962.
23. Redding, J. S.: Treatment of near drowning. *Int Anesth Clin, 3*:355-365, 1965.
24. Swann, H. G.: Studies in Resuscitation. Mem. Rep. Aero M. Lab. (MCREXD-696-79J) U.S. Air Force (no. 6006) pp. 1-74, October, 1950.
25. Banting, F. G.; Hall, G. E.; Janes, J. M.; Leibel, B., and Lougheed, D. W.: Physiological studies in experimental drowning (A preliminary report). *Canad Med Ass J, 39*:226-228, 1938.
26. Swann, H. G.: Studies in Resuscitation. U. S. Air Force Technical Report No. 6696. pp. 1-35, December, 1952.
27. Spitz, W. U., and Blanke, R. V.: Mechanism of death in fresh-water drowning. I. An experimental approach to the problem. *Arch Path (Chicago), 71*:661-668, 1961.

28. Gordon, A. S.; Ramon, F., and Ivy, A. C.: Drowning phenomena in various species. *Fed Proc, 13*:58, 1954.
29. Dumitru, A. P., and Hamilton, F. G.: A mechanism of drowning. *Anesth Analg (Cleveland), 42*:170-176, 1963.
30. Munroe, W. D.: Hemoglobinuria from near-drowning. *J Pediat, 64*:57-62, 1964.
31. Modell, J. H.: Resuscitation after aspiration of chlorinated fresh water. *JAMA, 185*:651-655, 1963.
32. Fainer, D. C.; Martin, C. G., and Ivy, A. C.: Resuscitation of dogs from fresh water drowning. *J Appl Physiol, 3*:417-426, 1951.

Chapter IX

NEUROLOGIC EFFECTS

T HERE ARE A NUMBER OF REPORTS in the literature of neurologic abnormalities following near-drowning. Prolonged unconsciousness with subsequent recovery,[1-5] blindness,[1] electroencephalographic changes,[5-7] dilatation of the ventricles suggesting brain atrophy,[1,5] and persistent coma until death[8,9] have all occurred.

Almost all victims of near-drowning suffer a period of unconsciousness, probably due to cerebral hypoxia. In a series of 29 consecutive near-drowning victims, all patients regained consciousness when normal levels of arterial oxygen tension and pH were reestablished. The four patients in this series, who eventually died, initially regained consciousness and remained conscious until adequate levels of arterial oxygen tension could no longer be maintained due to extensive intrapulmonary damage. None of the survivors had a demonstrable neurologic deficit.[10] Fuller reported 18 patients who suffered delayed death after near-drowning; 13 of these patients regained consciousness. At autopsy, two of his patients had laminar necrosis of the deep layers of the cerebral and cerebellar cortex, one had cerebral swelling with necrosis, and a fourth died with swelling and herniation.[4] Courville[8,9] has also reported necropsy findings compatible with cerebral anoxia in drowning victims.

It is of interest that, in neither Fuller's[4] nor Courville's[8,9] patients, where unconsciousness persisted or where unconsciousness or neurologic damage recurred after a lucid interval, was arterial blood analyzed for oxygen and carbon dioxide tensions or for pH. We are unable, therefore, to evaluate whether it was the near-drowning episode per se or the resultant hypoxia which led to the neurological changes in these patients. While changes in brain size due to acute hyper- or hypovolemia and electrolyte changes could contribute to the initial neurologic insult, this is unlikely since some of these patients had normal serum electrolyte concentrations. The most likely explanation is cerebral hypoxia due to inadequate oxygenation. Since determinations of arterial blood gas tensions and pH are now commonplace in most hospitals, it will be interesting to see if further cases of recurrent unconsciousness after resuscitation from near-drowning will be reported in the absence of hypoxemia. To date, none have been reported.

This question is frequently asked: How long can a patient be submerged and still be resuscitated? Monographs on resuscitation from sudden death[11] lead one to believe that biological death occurs within three to five minutes. There are reports in the literature, however, of patients resuscitated after submersion in fresh water for ten,[2] twenty[2] and twenty-two minutes,[1] and in tidal water for seventeen minutes.[3] The patient who was submerged for twenty-two minutes was rescued from a partially frozen river. Six hours after rescue, his body temperature was only 24°C. The other three patients were also hypothermic with temperatures ranging from 27°C to 32°C. The three victims of fresh water near-drowning developed prolonged neurologic deficits. Approximately one year later, however, they could all "function" normally, although some neurologic deficit was still present.[1,2] The patient rescued from tidal water is reported to have regained normal cerebral function twenty-six days after his accident.[3] Undoubtedly, the hypothermia was instrumental in the survival of all four of these patients. Gray[12] has demonstrated that hypothermia prolongs survival of rats during submersion in fresh water. He found that for every 5°C drop in temperature, survival was prolonged for ten seconds. This is not enough, however, to explain these seemingly miraculous recoveries. In light of these cases of successful resuscitation after prolonged submersion, one should not use time of submersion as the sole criterion for whether or not resuscitative efforts should be applied to a drowning victim.

Summary

The neurologic changes which occur during near-drowning and drowning are most likely due to the acute asphyxia and persistent hypoxia that results. When hypoxia and acidosis were corrected immediately, persistent coma and other neurologic deficits have not been reported. Since some patients have recovered after prolonged submersion, time alone should not be a determinant of whether or not resuscitative efforts should be started or continued on a drowning victim.

REFERENCES

1. Kvittingen, T. D., and Naess, A.: Recovery from drowning in fresh water. *Brit Med J, 5341*:1315-1317, 1963.
2. Ohlsson, K., and Beckman, M.: Drowning—reflections based on two cases. *Acta Chir Scand, 128*:327-339, 1964.
3. King, R. B., and Webster, I. W.: A case of recovery from drowning and prolonged anoxia. *Med J Aust, 1*:919-920, 1964.
4. Fuller, R. H.: The 1962 Wellcome prize essay. Drowning and the post-immersion syndrome. A clinicopathologic study. *Milit Med, 128*:22-36, 1963.
5. Odawara, M.; Haruna, H., and Fukuyama, Y.: Neurological sequelae after near-drowning. *Paediat Univ Tokyo, 11*:54-62, 1965.
6. Rath, C. E.: Drowning hemoglobinuria. *Blood, 8*:1099-1104, 1953.
7. Munroe, W. D.: Hemoglobinuria from near-drowning. *J Pediat, 64*:57-62, 1964.
8. Courville, C. B.: Case studies in cerebral anoxia. X. Effects of drowning on the brain observed after survival for six days. *Bull Los Angeles Neurol Soc, 20*:189-192, 1955.
9. Courville, C. B.: Anoxic changes in the brain after prolonged immersion. Report of a case with survival for nineteen days. *Bull Los Angeles Neurol Soc, 25*:165-169, 1960.
10. Butt, M. P.; Jalowayski, A.; Modell, J. H., and Giammona, S. T.: Pulmonary function after resuscitation from near-drowning. *Anesthesiology, 32*:275-277, 1970.
11. Jude, J. R., and Elam, J. O.: *Fundamentals of Cardiopulmonary Resuscitation.* Philadelphia, Davis, 1965.
12. Gray, S. W.: Respiratory movements of rat during drowning and influence of water temperature upon survival after submersion. *Amer J Physiol, 167*:95-102, 1951.

Chapter X

RENAL EFFECTS

W<small>HILE ADEQUATE RENAL FUNCTION</small> remains intact in most patients resuscitated after near-drowning, definite compromise of renal function has been reported. Fuller[1] found that 12 out of 50 victims of near-drowning had albuminuria, cylindruria, or both some time after their near-drowning episode. Hemoglobinuria has been reported to occur after near-drowning in fresh water[1-6] and salt water.[1] Oliguria and anuria can occur,[2,7] and in the most severe cases, renal damage may progress to acute tubular necrosis.[1]

Hemoglobinuria in these patients is associated with hemolysis. Albuminuria and anuria are not limited, however, to patients in whom hemolysis occurs.[7] This suggests that some patients may develop acute tubular necrosis secondary to a severe lactic acidosis and/or hypoxia. This author has seen one patient who maintained an adequate renal output and a clear urine, as long as her arterial oxygen tension was maintained above approximately 60 torr. When her PaO_2 fell below this value, oliguria and hematuria were present on repeated occasions.

Farthmann and Davidson[8] studied changes in renal function in dogs after near-drowning in fresh water. Of the 17 animals they studied, anuria occurred in five, and in 12 the urine was dark red. Out of these 17 animals, reestablishment and maintenance of tubular function could only be documented in five. Autopsy findings were not reported, however.

Summary

Evidence of renal damage is not a common finding after near-drowning. However, hemoglobinuria, hematuria, albuminuria, cylindruria, and anuria all can occur. In some very severe cases, acute tubular necrosis has occurred. Hemoglobinuria, hypoxia, and lactic acidosis have all been implicated as possible etiologic factors.

At present, hypoxia and metabolic acidosis must be regarded as the most likely causes for these abnormalities of renal function.

REFERENCES

1. Fuller, R. H.: The 1962 Wellcome prize essay. Drowning and the post-immersion syndrome. A clinicopathologic study. *Milit Med, 128*:22-36, 1963.
2. Kvittingen, T. D., and Naess, A.: Recovery from drowning in fresh water. *Brit Med J, 5341*:1315-1317, 1963.
3. Rath, C. E.: Drowning hemoglobinuria. *Blood, 8*:1099-1104, 1953.
4. Munroe, W. D.: Hemoglobinuria from near-drowning. *J Pediat, 64*:57-62, 1964.
5. King, R. B., and Webster, I. W.: A case of recovery from drowning and prolonged anoxia. *Med J Aust, 1*:919-920, 1964.
6. Redding, J. S., and Pearson, J. W.: Management of drowning victims. *GP, 29*:100-104, 1964.
7. Gambino, S. R: Personal communication. January 13, 1969.
8. Farthmann, E. H., and Davidson, A. I. G.: Fresh water drowning at lowered body temperature; an experimental study. *Amer J Surg, 109*:410-415, 1965.

Chapter XI

AUTOPSY FINDINGS IN VICTIMS OF DROWNING

JOSEPH H. DAVIS

THE FORENSIC PATHOLOGIST who investigates a death by drowning is faced with a number of problems. The first is to determine if the victim drowned. The complicating role of other diseases and chemicals needs to be determined. The manner of death—accident, suicide, or homicide—awaits clarification. Not to be ignored are public health considerations pertaining to a safer environment and better methods of therapy for the patient who has been submerged or near-drowned. Inasmuch as water covers the major part of the surface of the earth, contains innumerable varieties of animal life, and is occupied by diverse man-made vehicles, there appears to be unlimited opportunity for variable circumstances of injury and death. Drownings occur in oceans, bays, pools, rivers, lakes, industrial plants, bathtubs, deep water, shallow water, fresh water, sea water, clean and dirty water. The young and the elderly, the sick and the healthy, the drunk and the sober, swimmers and nonswimmers, boaters, and occupants of automobiles all may be involved in the interplay of man and his aquatic environment.

Because of the extreme variability of circumstances and patterns of drownings, one must consider drowning in the simplest of terms and use each individual circumstance to further qualify the case under investigation. In its barest essential, drowning is death due to submersion. Superimposed upon this simplistic definition are those variable findings associated with the nonuniform circumstances under which a victim drowns.

Investigation of a death suspected of drowning must include a consideration of the history, autopsy, and laboratory findings. Each must be considered in relation to the other, and the case must be considered as a whole. All too frequently, an investigator attempts to draw conclusions based upon a limited, noncorrelative approach. Eighty percent of all accidental deaths by drowning in the United States are classified as such without benefit of autopsy or laboratory findings. Obviously, those who are satisfied with a diagnosis of death by drowning based solely upon the history are content with shoddy investigations. On the other hand, a pathologist who performs autopsies or laboratory tests without regard for the circumstantial evidence may miss part of the overall picture as well.

The role of the medical investigator in an alleged case of drowning is to determine the cause of death, to participate in the classification of the manner of death (e.g. accident, suicide, homicide, and contribution by natural disease), and to anticipate future questions or allegations, thus, expanding the investigation to provide answers for these questions. Finally, the medical investigation should be concerned with obtaining data that can be used to improve treatment of future victims and to prevent needless deaths.

Since the inception of the medical examiner's office of Dade County (Miami), Florida, in 1956, there has been an average of 88 drownings per year. Approximately 14 percent involve children under five years of age. Motor vehicles entering the water account for 17 percent of the total. Suicides constitute 11 percent. Homicides are negligible; less than one percent. These drownings occur in a community of 1.3 million people residing in an area with 225 miles of canals, 75 rockpits, and 65 miles of bayfront. It is from study of these 88 annual cases, almost all subject to autopsy, that most of the autopsy and laboratory conclusions of this chapter are based.

EVIDENCE SURROUNDING THE DROWNING INCIDENT

The autopsy should be approached with an initial consideration of ancillary evidence to be examined. One must account for the condition of the clothing and the presence or absence of foreign matter such as mud, sand, or fuel. Postmortem injuries from sand, rocks, barnacles, boat propellors and postmortem resuscitative attempts should be recognized and documented. Occasionally, a question may arise as to the role of invertebrate stings in the production of incapacitation which leads to drowning. If agonal, such stings may not always produce skin lesions on the victim. In this instance, the microscopic-sized stinging nematocysts present upon the skin may be readily appreciated by rubbing one's forearm upon the surface of the body of the victim.[1]

Chemical intoxications, which play a role in initial carelessness and subsequent inability to be rescued, also should be considered. The foremost offender is alcohol, the ubiquitous catalyst found in a major percentage of all violent deaths. It is our experience that blood levels between 0.05 to 0.15 gm% of alcohol cause carelessness which can lead to water accidents. However, the victim usually attempts some reasonable effort at survival. When the blood level is 0.15 to 0.30 gm%, self-rescue attempts are less effectual. Over 0.30 gm%, the victim is often motionless and sufficiently anesthetized as to appear to have lost nervous reflexes and to be totally unaware that he no longer is breathing air.

In addition to alcohol, carbon monoxide must be considered when motor operated water vehicles are involved. Low blood levels, up to 10% hemoglobin saturation, can be due to cigarette smoking. Motor boating fatalities should always be examined for carbon monoxide, the source of which could be gasoline engine exhaust. A snorkeling free diver being towed at the surface behind a motor boat can become intoxicated with carbon monoxide. With self-contained underwater breathing apparatus (scuba), the victim may be unfortunate enough to have acquired a tank of air contaminated with carbon monoxide due to the use of an oil-contaminated air compressor. Aside from carbon monoxide, there also remains the possibility of a compressed air tank rusting, thus using up oxygen and leaving behind the nitrogen.

Drugs of all types may be encountered. Drowning while under the influence of hallucinogens, inhalable solvents, sedatives, stimulants, and narcotics is being seen with increasing frequency. Sudden, impulsive plunging into the water is of serious concern when young teenagers inhale glues and other solvents at the water's edge. Suicidal victims can be found with any variety of toxins within the stomach, more often than not a sedative. The presence of diphenylhydantoin and phenobarbital suggest the victim may have been an epileptic. Gingival hyperplasia, in the absence of therapeutic levels of the antiepileptic drugs, may suggest the victim had a seizure while swimming.

Often puzzling are those deaths which occur in athletic, sober, excellent swimmers who engage in underwater swimming while breath-holding. Under such circumstances, syncope may ensue and lead to a fatal outcome.[2,3]

In summation, the investigation of a water death must rest upon a total integration of circumstantial evidence, autopsy, and laboratory findings. Laboratory tests must be guided by individual consideration and interpreted accordingly.

AUTOPSY FINDINGS

While much has been written about the autopsy evidence of drowning, there has been little emphasis upon the variability of autopsy findings. For all practical purposes, the autopsy findings in death due to drowning cannot be described in consistent terms.

Cutis anserina, or goose flesh, may be present; but this is not related to water submersion as much as it is to the contraction of the erector pili muscles from any mechanical stimulus with rigor holding them in the contracted position. Water wrinkling of the thick skin of the hands and feet may appear after several hours, especially in hypertonic ocean water. This finding is not dependent upon the cause of death but only indicates that the body was in the water. Pale or sanguineous watery foam from the nose and mouth is a most frequent finding. Mud and aquatic debris may be admixed. Often vomitus is present. The eyes are usually not remarkable, although the exposed bulbar conjunctivae may reveal a brownish discoloration as it dries; particularly after sea water exposure.

The mouth and upper airway often contain, in addition to foam and vomitus, aquatic plants, sand, or other material if the water is impure. Under such circumstances, the penetration of fluid into the air passages, paranasal sinuses, and middle ears may be demonstrated at the autopsy table. Gardner[4] cites an instance of a two and one-half year-old boy who fell head first into an oil drum containing six inches of chalk and soot-contaminated water. The sooty material could be traced easily to a point about an inch below the vocal cords, indicating that deeper aspiration of the water did not take place in this instance. In our experience, we have always been able to trace grossly visible particulate matter into deeper air passages if the mouth contained foreign material.

Upon opening the pleura, the lungs are usually found to be voluminous and may approach each other in the anterior midline. The lungs neither collapse when the pleural space is opened nor contract readily when cut and, in this effect, may resemble lungs from an asthmatic. This is best demonstrated in the elastic undamaged lungs of a child as compared with the sodden, often tobacco-stained lungs of the drowned, older adult. The lungs appear irregularly congested with some degree of pink-red mottling. The coloration and degree of entrapment of air in the periphery is variable. Usually, the lungs of a child have more distention by entrapped air than those of elderly adults. On cut section, watery fluid tends to pour forth in the latter instance as compared with the former, where pressure produces a fine bubbling of sanguineous watery foam from transected air passages. The lungs from a drowned child might appear unusually dry to an inexperienced observer and could thus lead to an erroneous conclusion that there was no aspiration of water.

The pleural spaces are moist with variable quantities of light straw-colored fluid, usually only a few milliliters in quantity. As the postmortem interval increases, autolysis and putrefaction occur. The lungs then may collapse and the pleural space become occupied by several hundred milliliters of almost black, foul, watery fluid upon which floats small globules of liquefied body fat. Unless the victim had a prior pleural effusion, this represents transudation of fluid from the edematous lung. Microscopic sections of lung tissue may disclose variable degrees of alveolar distention, edematous protein precipitate, and focal intra-alveolar hemorrhage. Fuller[5] has described agglutinated platelets in pulmonary vessels and speculated upon their relationship to fluid blood which is usually observed in the great vessels at autopsy. It might be noted, however, that postmortem fibrin clots may be prominent in a drowned individual who has had a prior infection, malignancy, or other necrotic lesion. Similarly, an individual with sickle cell phenotype may have copious amounts of dark clots, particularly between the trabeculae carneae of the cardiac ventricles.

The stomach may contain swallowed fluid. On occasion, ingested fluid passes through the pylorus into the small intestine. The liver, spleen, and kidneys may appear acutely congested. The brain, particularly in a child, becomes moderately swollen. In many cases, cyanosis of the cortex is quite striking particularly when the cut surface of the cerebellar cortex is observed.

Although it has been known for many years that the middle ears may contain drowning fluid,[6] there has been recent emphasis upon hemorrhage in the middle ears and mastoids in drowning.[7] Niles[8] demonstrated this in 23 of 24 cases of drowning and 18 of 25 cases of possible drowning, the latter category not being further clarified. We frequently have observed middle ear hemorrhage and find it a helpful sign. One must be careful, however, to avoid confusing autolysis and postmortem dependent lividity stasis with an acute hemorrhage. Visual inspection of the middle ear cavity after removing the cortical bone is the easiest technique used to demonstrate this phenomenon. In drowning, one usually sees a little sanguineous moisture or fluid in the middle ears. Although one may speculate as to the origin of bloody fluid in the middle ear, it seems most reasonable that violent struggling in conjunction with water pressure can exert positive and negative pressures upon the fragile capillaries of the mucous membrane, thus leading to extravasation of blood into the moist fluid. A plugged eustachian tube can prevent the pressure transmittal and spare the middle ear from hemorrhage as was noted in the case of a two year-old infant who fell into a canal of fresh water, struggled upon the surface, floated quietly for a short time, and then sank to the bottom in twelve feet of water. Only the left middle ear and surrounding air spaces contained sanguineous moisture. The right middle ear was pale and contained mucopurulent exudate.

DELAYED DEATH AFTER NEAR-DROWNING

The pathological findings after delayed death in near-drowning cases are varied. If the victim was anoxic for a sufficient length of time, the brain will show lesions of anoxic degeneration. The exact gross and microscopic changes seen will vary with the degree and duration of cerebral anoxia. Rapid death, within a few hours or days, may reveal gross changes only of swelling. Later, anoxic perivascular hemorrhages may be seen. Within a week or two, basal ganglia or midbrain cystic degenerations may appear. These findings are not unique to drowning, but are those of nonspecific anoxia.[9] An autopsy surgeon should beware of embalming artefact which may be superimposed upon a softened anoxic brain. Under such circumstances, pressurized injections of embalming fluid may force softened cerebellum into the foramen magnum, leading one to suspect antemortem swelling of a greater degree than was present. This same artefact may be seen if the victim drowns, the body is not recovered until partially autolyzed, and then is energetically embalmed prior to autopsy.

The other common pathway of death after apparent near-drowning is due to irreversible pulmonary damage. The changes in the lungs vary according to the length of survival, whether or not aspiration of water, foreign matter, or gastric juice has occurred, and whether or not secondary infection with bacteria takes place. Added to this may be the lesions of pulmonary oxygen toxicity when high inspired oxygen tensions are necessary during therapy for prolonged periods of time.[10] In those patients who die of pulmonary edema fairly soon after live rescue from clean water, the autopsy lung findings may be the same as those in a nonrevived drowning victim. With longer time intervals, gross and microscopic evidence of pneumonitis becomes pronounced.[5,11] For example, in two cases, reported in more detail elsewhere,[12] one victim survived 18 hours and the other 85 hours after rescue. The first, a six-year-old boy, was neither apneic nor unconscious immediately after rescue from sea water. He survived for 18 hours. During hospitalization he experienced progressive dyspnea and lost consciousness. At autopsy, the entire right lung, and most of the left, had an increased consistency and a red-brown-purple color. Pinkish frothy fluid could be expressed from the lower airway and cut surface of the lung. Microscopic sections revealed a diffuse intra-alveolar pink, finely granular deposit of proteinaceous edema fluid. Thin, pink hyaline membranes were prominent within alveoli and thicker membranes were seen in the alveolar ducts. Variable intra-alveolar hemorrhages were present. Less prominent were occasional areas of peribronchiolar interstitial and intra-alveolar infiltration.

The second case was that of a 14-year-old girl who was trapped on the bottom of a fresh water swimming pool for approximately ten minutes before rescue. She was unconscious and apneic when rescued. Her condition was precarious and, although conciousness returned, adequate respiratory function could not be reestablished. She died 85 hours after admission. At autopsy, there was approximately 500 ml of thick, dark proteinaceous fluid within each pleural space. Fibrinous pleural exudate was present, particularly on the lower lobe of the right lung. Cut sections of each lung were dark purple in color and had a nodular consistency. The lungs were almost devoid of air. Pressure produced a thick, semi-mucoid, slightly purulent exudate from the surface. Microscopic sections revealed no normal parenchyma or any well-aerated sections. There were diffuse hyaline membranes lining the alveoli and alveolar ducts throughout all sections. Some alveoli contained a light pink proteinaceous exudate. Scattered intra-alveolar hemorrhages were present. Neutrophilic exudate was scant. The intralobular septa were edematous and focally infiltrated by lymphocytes, monocytes, and a few neutrophiles. The bronchiolar epithelium was focally ulcerated and the exposed submucosa was heavily infiltrated with neutrophils and monocytic cells. An occasional bronchiole contained a small fragment of aspirated vegetable matter. Focal areas of necrosis of the alveolar septa were present. In these areas, bacterial clusters were prominent.

Summary

The autopsy findings of the postimmersion syndrome appear to be mainly confined to the brain and lung. The changes depend, to a great extent, upon the duration of survival, the initial degree of apnea, the effects of aspirated fluid, the length and severity of hypoxia, and the effects of therapy. The pulmonary changes are primarily those of an initial chemical pneumonitis instead of a bacterial infection.

REFERENCES

1. Ioannides, G., and Davis, J. H.: Portuguese man-of-war stinging. *Arch Derm, 91*:448-451, 1965.
2. Davis, J. H.: Fatal underwater breath holding in trained swimmers. *J Forensic Sci, 6*:301-306, 1961.
3. Craig, A. B., Jr.: Causes of loss of consciousness during underwater swimming. *J Appl Physiol, 16*:583-586, 1961.
4. Gardner, E.: Mechanism of certain forms of sudden death in medico-legal practice. *Med Legal Criminol Rev, 10*:120-133, 1942.
5. Fuller, R. H.: The 1962 Wellcome prize essay. Drowning and the post-

immersion syndrome. A clinicopathological study. *Milit Med, 128*: 22-36, 1963.

6. Hough, G. de N.: The post-mortem signs of drowning. *Boston M & S J, 133*:409-412, 1895.

7. Mueller, W. F.: Pathology of temporal bone hemorrhage in drowning. *J Forensic Sci, 14*:327-336, 1969.

8. Niles, N. R.: Hemorrhage in the middle-ear and mastoid in drowning. *Amer J Clin Path, 40*:281-283, 1963.

9. Courville, C. B.: *Contributions to the Study of Cerebral Anoxia.* Los Angeles, San Lucas Press, 1953.

10. Nash, G.; Blennerhassett, J. B., and Pontoppidan, H.: Pulmonary lesions associated with oxygen therapy and artificial ventilation. *New Eng J Med, 276*:368-374, 1967.

11. Fuller, R. H.: The clinical pathology of human near-drowning. *Proc Roy Soc Med, 56*:33-38, 1963.

12. Modell, J. H.; Davis, J. H.; Giammona, S. T.; Moya, F., and Mann, J. B.: Blood gas and electrolyte changes in human near-drowning victims. *JAMA, 203*:337-343, 1968.

Chapter XII

TESTS FOR DROWNING

JOSEPH H. DAVIS

A NEVER-ENDING SEARCH for a "drowning test" pervades the literature. That this will-o'-the-wisp shall never be obtained is to be expected in view of the variability of drowning circumstances discussed in Chapter XI. The literature, extending back a century, takes cognizance of the variable amounts of water which may be aspirated during drowning. Laryngeal spasms, prior physical condition, intoxication, and autonomic nervous system reflexes all may be expected to play a role in the rapidity of death, the volume of water aspirated, and the resulting autopsy findings. Basically, the "drowning tests" are but a search for evidence of aspiration of water. The theory is that blood on the left side of the heart becomes diluted by the aspirated fluid. Evidence of such is sought on the basis of simple dilution,[1] specific gravity changes,[2] or by the concentration of chlorides or magnesium. Finally, there remains the hope that diatoms, aspirated in the agonal moments, can be detected elsewhere in the body as evidence of aspiration of fluid. None of these tests suffice to establish or rule out drowning. For example, if the victim dies while submerged, but does not aspirate water, the above tests are worthless. These so-called drowning tests are no more diagnostic of drowning than a single blood glucose determination is exclusively diagnostic of diabetes mellitus.

In 1921, Gettler first proposed a method for the determination of death by drowning based upon the differences of the chloride content in the right and left side of the heart.[3] Since then, the "Gettler test" has achieved widespread acceptance. However, as early as 1925, Palmer and Doherty[4] expressed some doubt as to the original conclusions. Thirteen years later, Palmer[5] felt that the test was of more value in salt water drowning than in fresh water drowning. Moritz, in 1944,[6] reviewed all the chemical methods that had been advocated to determine death from drowning. He pointed out the variation of blood chloride concentration which occurred as a function of the postmortem interval alone. Magnesium, as an indicator of aspiration of sea water, was considered. Nondrowned dogs showed differences in right and left heart magnesium during the postmortem interval which increased as decomposition advanced. With salt water drowning, a pronounced increase in magnesium on the left, as compared with the right, might constitute presumptive evidence of aspiration of sea water. Bowden later reported[7] five sea water drownings, in which four of these had pronounced increases in magnesium in the left as compared with the right. However, the one case without change was not discussed in detail. Durlacher, Freimuth, and Swann[2] concluded that the plasma specific gravity difference between the two sides of the heart was more reliable than the chloride change. In a series of 118 consecutive drowning victims, Modell and Davis[8] found the specific gravity of plasma to be less in the left ventricle than in the right in 91 percent of fresh water drownings, 79 percent of salt water drowning victims, and 75 percent of nondrowned persons.

As an extension of the observed aspiration of particulate matter in many drowning victims, there has been considerable interest in the significance of diatoms which may be found in the lungs and in more remote viscera of the body. Thomas, Van Hecke, and Timperman[9] reviewed their experiences and those of others, and felt that such formed elements would be of great diagnostic value in suspected death by drowning. Spitz and Schneider[10] found that air contamination could lead to diatoms in tissues of nondrowned persons. Neidhart and Greendyke,[11] reporting from upstate New York, felt that nonrespiratory visceral demonstration of diatoms would be significant of aspiration of contaminated water because the air and the drinking water are not normally contaminated in their area remote from the sea. A point not considered by them is that diatomaceous earth filters are quite common for home swimming pools. Persons swallowing such water could conceivably acquire diatoms in viscera, and then subsequently die of causes other than drowning. As with all tests, the interpretation must include the full realization of all possible variables for that particular place and time.

Summary

The so-called "drowning tests" do not exist as such. Individuals drown in such variable fashions and circumstances as to prevent the unqualified interpretation of a diagnostic "drowning test." Those tests, based upon a difference between components of the left and right side of the heart, rest upon the assumption that the last gasp with aspiration of water occurred almost simultaneously with cessation of heartbeat so that the postmortem chemistries are indicative of this exact circumstance. But what of the panic-stricken boy who is pulled from the water, whose last gasp may be air instead of water, and whose heartbeat continues for a few more minutes? What of those individuals who inhale small quantities of water? Data from human drowning victims indicates that approximately 85 percent of both fresh and sea water drowning victims aspirate 22 ml or less of water per kilogram of body weight.[8] It would appear that there are no pathognomonic "drowning tests." Laboratory tests applied to cases of suspected drowning must be utilized only with the understanding that they are subject to wide variations of results and cannot be accepted on face value.

REFERENCES

1. Chiaraviglio, E. del C., and Wolf, A. V.: Diagnosis of drowning. *Arch Path, 75*:337-341, 1963.
2. Durlacher, S. H.; Freimuth, H. C., and Swann, H. E., Jr.: Blood changes in man following death due to drowning, with comments on tests for drowning. *AMA Arch Path, 56*:454-461, 1953.
3. Gettler, A. O.: A method for the determination of death by drowning. *JAMA, 77*:1650-1652, 1921.
4. Palmer, A. A., and Doherty, W. M.: A method for the determination of death by drowning. *Med J Aust, 2*:103-104, 1925.
5. Palmer, A.: Gettler's test in cases of drowning. *Med J Aust, 2*:129, 1938.
6. Moritz, A. R.: Chemical methods for the determination of death by drowning. *Physiol Rev, 24*:70-88, 1944.
7. Bowden, K.: Drowning. *Med J Aust, 1*:39-43, 1957.
8. Modell, J. H., and Davis, J. H.: Electrolyte changes in human drowning victims. *Anesthesiology, 30*:414-420, 1969.
9. Thomas, F.; Van Hecke, W., and Timperman, J.: The medicolegal diagnosis of death by drowning. *J Forensic Sci, 8*:1-14, 1963.

10. Spitz, W. U., and Schneider, V.: The significance of diatoms in the diagnosis of death by drowning. *J Forensic Sci, 9*:11-18, 1964.
11. Neidhart, D. A., and Greendyke, R. M.: The significance of diatom demonstration in the diagnosis of death by drowning. *Amer J Clin Path, 48*:377-382, 1967.

Chapter XIII

RETRIEVAL AND ACUTE THERAPY

T HE PRIME OBJECTIVE *of emergency therapy for the near-drowning victim is to restore normal arterial blood gas and acid-base levels by effective ventilation, circulation, oxygenation, and the judicious use of buffers.*

RESCUE

The near-drowning victim should be maintained in a position which permits emergency resuscitative measures to be performed as soon as he has been rescued. As early as 1796, a number of hooks, boats, floating stretchers, and other devices were proposed for aiding in water rescue.[1] These and newer articles have recently been reviewed in pictorial form.[2] Most of the equipment used over the years was heavy and cumbersome. However, since styrofoam plastics are now available, it would seem reasonable that a lightweight, contoured, floatable stretcher might be constructed for rescue purposes. In most cases, appliances are unnecessary and would only cause delay in initiating resuscitation. In others, particularly when the rescuer is not an accomplised swimmer, it may be advantageous to have a means of external support for the patient. It should be emphasized, though, that since the degree of hypoxia increases rapidly with the duration of apnea, the use of a rescue stretcher must not delay the initiation of artificial ventilation.

VENTILATION

If the victim is apneic when rescued, treatment by artificial ventilation must begin immediately. Over the years, a number of methods for providing artificial ventilation have been used. The studies of Safar, Escarraga, and Elam[3] have shown that mouth-to-mouth ventilation produces more effective ventilation than the previously popular external chest compression methods. Mouth-to-mouth resuscitation is the only method that meets all the requirements of the ideal emergency ventilator. It is simple, portable, instantly available, reliable, and inexpensive. It has a self-contained power source and an inexhaustible oxygen supply. It fits all patients and the rate and volume of ventilation can be varied to match the needs of the victim.[4]

Effective mechanical ventilation is possible only if the victim has a patent airway. To provide an adequate airway, the patient's mouth should be opened, if possible, and the posterior pharynx rapidly inspected (both visually and by palpation) for foreign objects, secretions, vomitus, or other matter. Any material found is to be removed. Solid objects are best removed by hand. In the absence of mechanical suction equipment, emergency cleansing of secretions can be achieved by swabbing the mouth and hypopharynx with fingers wrapped in an absorbent material. Placing the head in maximum extension and lifting the jaw forward usually will produce a patent airway.

Then, the rescurer's mouth is placed over the victim's mouth and the rescuer uses his exhaled air to inflate the patient's lungs. Successful inflation is confirmed by observing that the patient's chest rises with each ventilatory attempt. If, for any reason, it is not possible to ventilate the victim's lungs by the mouth-to-mouth method, an attempt should be made to provide mouth-to-nose ventilation. If this also fails, the rescuer should recheck whether or not he has removed all foreign objects and provided maximum hyperextension of the patient's head and elevation of his jaw to establish a patent airway. Occasionally, placement of a mechanical aid, such as a nasopharyngeal airway, oropharyngeal airway, or an endotracheal tube may be necessary. It should be emphasized that endotracheal intubation usually is not necessary to provide a clear airway. Intubation should be attempted only after the patient has been reoxygenated and only by individuals skilled in such techniques. Similarly, tracheostomy is rarely indicated at this time. Merely placing a hole in the trachea does not provide adequate ventilation and oxygenation and the time lost during this procedure may be critical in determining the outcome of the resuscitation. It also has been clearly demonstrated that the incidence of complications when emergency tracheostomy is performed under adverse conditions is formidable.[5]

Attempting to drain water from the lungs of a victim of near-drowning in fresh water is a waste of time, since the aspirated water is absorbed very rapidly from the lung into the circulation.[6-13] During near-drowning in sea water, the hypertonic fluid draws plasma from the circulation into the lungs.[6-8,12,14,15] It may be possible to remove some of this fluid from the lungs by proper positioning of the patient to promote drainage. This must be done, however, without compromising artificial ventilation.

Near-drowning and drowning victims frequently swallow large quantities of water prior to losing consciousness. If a clear airway is not established during resuscitative efforts, air can be forced into the stomach producing further distention. Active or passive regurgitation may then take place. This is the most common origin of large quantities of fluid which may appear in the oropharynx during resuscitation attempts. Precautions must be taken to prevent aspiration of this liquid by its removal from the oropharynx. Time should not be wasted in attempting to drain the stomach during the acute phase of resuscitation; however, extreme care should be taken to avoid further gastric distention.

Near-drowning victims who have aspirated water will remain hypoxic, even though adequate volumes of air are moved during resuscitative attempts, unless supplemental oxygen is given. This is due to the intrapulmonary shunting which results from the aspirated fluid. For this reason, once the proper equipment is assembled and the rescuer is in a position to use it effectively mouth-to-mouth ventilation should be replaced by a method of intermittent positive pressure ventilation that is capable of supplying high inspired oxygen concentrations. Hand-operated or controlled units are preferable to automatic cycling devices. Most automatic devices are pressure-limited and in the face of a low compliance they can be cycled, or shut off, before effective volumes of gas are delivered. This is particularly true if the patient requires simultaneous ventilation of the lungs and maintenance of the circulation by closed chest cardiac massage, since the pressures generated on chest compression will cycle the ventilator.

If the patient breathes spontaneously after rescue or begins to breathe after a successful resuscitation attempt, the rescuer should not be lulled into a false sense of security. The highest available oxygen concentration must be delivered to the patient until quantitative measurements (PaO_2) have been made to determine that supplemental oxygen therapy is no longer needed.

If the victim falls into the *drown without aspiration* group, and effective circulation is still intact when breathing is reestablished, the probability of complete recovery from the asphyxial state is good.[16] If the duration of hypoxia is short, further therapy may not be necessary. If the patient has aspirated water, however, the pulmonary lesion is not as readily reversible. This makes the prognosis less favorable and further therapy is imperative. Since the rescuer cannot tell at the scene of the accident which patients have aspirated and which have not, it is imperative that all near-drowning victims be taken to the hospital for further evaluation and therapy.

CIRCULATION

As soon as mouth-to-mouth ventilation has been started, evidence of an effective circulation should be elicited by palpation of the carotid, radial, or femoral pulses. Fixed and dilated pupils can not be used as absolute criteria for circulatory arrest. Some patients will have small pupils in the face of circulatory arrest, while in the presence of profound hypoxia the pupils may be fixed and dilated even though circulation is still intact. If the presence of an effective heartbeat can not be verified by palpation of pulses or auscultation of heart sounds, the patient is judged to be in cardiovascular collapse or circulatory arrest, and closed chest cardiac massage must be added immediately to the ventilatory phase of resuscitation. This subject has been dealt with extensively in recent years and excellent monographs are available for a detailed description and discussion of the techniques.[17,18] Only the essential details will be outlined here.

To eject blood from the heart by external cardiac compression, the heel of one hand is placed over the lower third of the sternum. The heel of the other hand is placed on top of the first and the sternum is pushed downward toward the spine approximately 5 cm in adults. The sternum is held in this position for approximately one-half of a second and then released rapidly. This procedure should be repeated 60 to 80 times per minute. In small children it is necessary to compress the sternum with only one hand, while for infants, the tips of two fingers usually will suffice. The rate of massage in infants and children should be 100 to 120 times per minute, and the point of compression is the midsternum. The presence of a good carotid or femoral pulse each time the heart is massaged is presumptive evidence of effective circulation. Obviously, it requires a second rescuer to monitor one of these pulses.

It must be emphasized that external cardiac compression, alone, does not produce effective ventilation of the lungs. Therefore, it must be combined with mouth-to-mouth ventilation. This is done, to better advantage, by a second rescuer giving one artificial breath for every five chest compressions. If only one rescuer is present, he must do both mouth-to-mouth ventilation and closed chest cardiac massage. This is accomplished by alternating two quick lung inflations with fifteen sternal compressions. To the inexperienced rescurer, it should be emphasized that the ventilation is of primary importance and the mouth-to-mouth ventilation must not be compromised at any cost.

When circulatory arrest has occurred secondary to hypoxia, the artificial ventilation and circulation produced by mouth-to-mouth ventilation and closed chest cardiac massage may be sufficient to reoxygenate the myocardium and reestablish cardiac action. In some victims, effective myocardial action may not return immediately because of severe acidosis. In others, the heart may be in a state of ventricular fibrillation. The differentiation between asystole and ventricular fibrillation cannot be made without an electrocardiagram. In view of the fact that the emergency rescuer rarely has the equipment available to make this differentiation, he must continue mechanical ventilation and cardiac compression until a specific diagnosis is established and specific therapy is available. In some communities, the necessary equipment will be available in the rescue ambulance, but in most areas definitive diagnosis and treatment must wait until the patient reaches the hospital.

DRUGS

Oxygen is the most important drug for the treatment of a patient after near-drowning. Oxygen lack, or hypoxia, is the single most important cause of death and sequelae from drowning, regardless of the quantity or type of water aspirated, or the duration of immersion without aspiration.[9,10,14,19,20] Its supply is abundant, although at a borderline tension, in the ambient air, and supplemental sources to deliver higher oxygen concentrations are often available at public beaches and swimming pools. Oxygen can be administered without benefit of specialized equipment, e.g. needles and syringes. It should be delivered in the highest possible concentration as an adjuvant to, but not as a substitute for, effective ventilation in all near-drowning victims until determinations of the arterial oxygen tension are made in the hospital. Only then can it be established that supplemental oxygen is no longer required.

The second drug which should be considered in the emergency treatment of the near-drowning victim is *bicarbonate* or another buffer solution to correct the metabolic acidosis which so frequently accompanies hypoxia. We prefer to use sodium bicarbonate solution rather than buffers, such as THAM, because it is more readily available and knowledge of its use is more universal among physicians. While the use of either of these drugs would be desirable at the scene of an accident, the requirement for specialized equipment, *e.g.* needles and syringes, usually precludes their administration until the patient is admitted to the hospital. Respiratory stimulants, such as picrotoxin, Metrazol®, ammonia, caffeine, sodium benzoate, doxapram and others, as a rule are rarely effective and may cause serious side effects, notably cerebral hypoxia, vomiting, and convulsions. Therefore, they have no place in the therapy of the near-drowning victim.

Again, it should be emphasized that the prime objective of emergency therapy for the near-drowning victim is *to restore normal arterial blood gas and acid-base levels by effective ventilation, circulation, oxygenation and by judicious use of buffers.* The methods used to accomplish these objectives should be those most readily available and those proven to be most effective. Return of spontaneous ventilation or of consciousness is not a guarantee of survival. All patients, regardless of their condition after rescue, must be transported to the hospital for further evaluation and therapy. It should be obvious that treatment must continue en route from the scene of the accident to the hospital.

REFERENCES

1. Herholdt, J. D., and Rafn, C. G.: *An Attempt at an Historical Survey of Life-Saving Measures for Drowning Persons and Information of the Best Means by Which They Can Be Brought Back to Life.* Denmark, Aarhuus, Stiftsbogtrykkerie, 1960 (Copenhagen, H. Tikiob's, 1796).

2. Crosfill, J. W. L.: Drowning. *Proc Roy Soc Med, 49*:1051-1058, 1956.

3. Safar, P.; Escarraga, L. A., and Elam, J. O.: A comparison of the mouth-to-mouth and mouth-to-airway methods of artificial respiration with chest-pressure arm-lift methods. *New Eng J Med, 258*:671-677, 1958.

4. Modell, J. H.: Basic principles of acute and chronic respirator therapy. In Banyai, A. L. and Gordon, B. L.: *Advances in Cardiopulmonary Diseases.* Chicago, Year Bk Med, 1969, Vol. IV, pp. 225-248.

5. Yarington, C. T., Jr., and Frazer, J. P.: Complications of tracheotomy. *Arch Surg (Chicago), 91*:652-655, 1965.

6. Swann, H. G., and Spafford, N. R.: Body salt and water changes during fresh and sea water drowning. *Texas Rep Biol Med, 9*:356-382, 1951.

7. Swann, H. G., and Brucer, M.: The cardiorespiratory and biochemical events during rapid anoxic death. VI. Fresh water and sea water drowning. *Texas Rep Biol Med, 7*:604-618, 1949.

8. Swann, H. G.; Brucer, M.; Moore, C., and Vezien, B. L.: Fresh water and sea water drowning: A study of the terminal cardiac and biochemical events. *Texas Rep Biol Med, 5*:423-437, 1947.

9. Modell, J. H.; Gaub, M.; Moya, F.; Vestal, B., and Swarz, H.: Physiologic effects of near drowning with chlorinated fresh water, distilled water and isotonic saline. *Anesthesiology, 27*:33-41, 1966.

10. Modell, J. H., and Moya, F.: Effects of volume of aspirated fluid during chlorinated fresh water drowning. *Anesthesiology, 27*:662-672, 1966.

11. Redding, J. S., and Cozine, R. A.: Restoration of circulation after fresh water drowning. *J Appl Physiol, 16*:1071-1074, 1961.

12. Halmagyi, D. F. J.: Lung changes and incidence of respiratory arrest in rats after aspiration of sea and fresh water. *J Appl Physiol, 16*:41-44, 1961.

13. Reuben, A., and Reuben, H.: Artificial respiration. Flow of water from the lungs and the stomach. *Lancet, 1*:780-781, 1962.

14. Modell, J. H.; Moya, F.; Newby, E. J.; Ruiz, B. C., and Showers, A. V.: The effects of fluid volume in seawater drowning. *Ann Intern Med, 67*:68-80, 1967.

15. Redding, J. S.; Voigt, G. C., and Safar, P.: Treatment of sea-water aspiration. *J Appl Physiol, 15*:1113-1116, 1960.

16. Redding, J.; Voigt, G. C., and Safar, P.: Drowning treated with intermittent positive pressure breathing. *J Appl Physiol, 15*:849-854, 1960.

17. Jude, J. R., and Elam, J. O.: *Fundamentals of Cardiopulmonary Resuscitation.* Philadelphia, Davis, 1965.

18. Committee on Cardiopulmonary Resuscitation: *Cardiopulmonary Resuscitation. A Manual for Instructors.* American Heart Association, 1967.
19. Modell, J. H.; Davis, J. H.; Giammona, S. T.; Moya, F., and Mann, J B.: Blood gas and electrolyte changes in human near-drowning victims. *JAMA, 203*:337-343, 1968.
20. Modell, J. H.; Moya, F.; Williams, H. D., and Weibley, T. C.: Changes in blood gases and A-aDO$_2$ during near-drowning. *Anesthesiology, 29*:456-465, 1968.

Chapter XIV

HOSPITAL THERAPY

SINCE RETURN OF CONSCIOUSNESS after resuscitation from near-drowning is not synonymous with normal survival, and delayed sequelae or even death from hypoxia occurs,[1-3] all near-drowning victims should be admitted to the hospital. During transport, inhalation of oxygen should be continued regardless of the patient's apparent clinical condition, and ventilatory assistance should be provided when indicated.

Hospital therapy should initially be aimed at intensive pulmonary care. The extent of pulmonary care necessary will depend upon the condition of the individual patient. It may range from simple oxygen administration to establishing a patent airway with a cuffed endotracheal tube which, in turn, is connected to a mechanical ventilator for continuous ventilatory support. All near-drowning victims should receive 100% oxygen by inhalation until analysis of arterial blood for oxygen tension confirms it is no longer necessary. If ventilatory assistance is required, it should be provided first by controlling or assisting the patient's ventilation with a mask, nonrebreathing valve, and reservoir bag. Intubation of the trachea will be necessary in many of these patients to establish a suitable airway for providing prolonged mechanical ventilation. An endotracheal tube also provides a route for direct endotracheal suctioning, administration of drugs in aerosol form, and periodic hyperinflation of the lungs. Because of the hazards of hypoxia, intubation should be attempted only after reoxygenation and by physicians skilled in the technique. Emergency tracheostomy rarely is indicated since an adequate airway usually can be provided via the orotracheal or nasotracheal route.

In this author's experience, approximately 80 percent of near-drowning victims had some degree of metabolic acidosis accompanying their hypoxia (Chap. III). In many, it was profound (pHa

< 7.10). It is recommended, therefore, that sodium bicarbonate (0.3 to 0.4 mEq/lb of body weight) be administered intravenously, on an empirical basis, to all near-drowning victims as soon as they are brought to the emergency room. If the patient happens not to have acidemia, it is unlikely that the mild alkalemia that results from this treatment would have any deleterious effect. As soon as possible, of course, arterial blood should be drawn for determination of pH, Po_2, Pco_2 and bicarbonate. The extent of ventilatory support, the inspired oxygen concentration, and further bicarbonate administration necessary to produce normal carbon dioxide elimination, oxygenation, and acid-base balance respectively will be determined by these values. A microhematocrit determination should also be made. Unless obvious hemolysis or a markedly abnormal hematocrit are seen, significant fluid or electrolyte disturbances are unlikely,[2,4-6] and the problems in treating the patient will be related almost exclusively to ventilation, oxygenation, and acid-base balance.

If bronchospasm is present from aspiration of fluid,[7] it can be treated by administration of an aerosol of a bronchodilating agent such as isoproterenol. Pulmonary edema frequently is seen after near-drowning with aspiration.[8] Some patients present with pink froth or foam in the mouth and nose, while in others the "gurgling" of pulmonary edema is heard only with the stethoscope. Nebulized 20% to 30% ethyl alcohol will be helpful in changing the surface tension of these bubbles.[9] When the surface tension of the bubbles no longer can change with size, they cannot maintain their integrity. The bubbles rupture and, therefore, the mechanical blocking to ventilation of the airway is reduced.

Active measures should also be taken to reinflate atelectatic alveoli by frequent hyperinflation with positive pressure. While this can be done automatically at set intervals with certain IPPB devices, it is achieved more reliably by an experienced person using a simple system consisting of a large anesthesia bag and nonrebreathing valve connected directly to the endotracheal tube. This method provides the added advantage of "feeling" the patient's compliance and comparing it from one treatment period to another. Depending upon the patient, hyperinflation treatment may be necessary as frequently as every ten minutes or only every few hours.

If the patient's arterial oxygen tension is below 80 torr (at FIO_2 = .21), it suggests that he has aspirated fluid and he should be treated prophylactically for aspiration pneumonitis with broad spectrum antibiotics and steroids.[10,11] There is little evidence to support the use of one steroid over another or, for that matter, one dosage over another. A routine followed in many clinics is Hydrocortone® sodium succinate, 100 mg I.V. or I.M. every 6 hours during the acute stage. Equivalent doses of other steroid preparations are apparently as effective clinically. Steroids may be discontinued once a consistent trend of an increasing PaO_2 is observed. If steroids have been given for at least five days, they should be withdrawn gradually by progressively decreasing the dosage. If a shorter course of therapy was given, "tapering" usually is unnecessary.

Many patients vomit, either during the near-drowning episode or while emergency resuscitation is attempted, and they may aspirate solid debris or particles of undigested food. Serial physical and radiographic examination of the chest will prove helpful in diagnosing airway obstruction from aspirated material. A case illustrating this point follows:

Case 1

This seven-year-old child was found floating face down in a fresh water swimming pool. He was apneic when rescued, and although his pupils were fixed and dilated, a pulse was still palpable. He was treated with mouth-to-mouth resuscitation at poolside. During the resuscitation procedure, the patient vomited. Spontaneous ventilation returned and he was rushed to the hospital.

On admission to the hospital, he was deeply cyanotic and there was pink frothy foam coming out of his mouth and nose. While he breathed 40% oxygen the pH of his arterial blood was 7.03, PaO_2 was 58 torr, $PaCO_2$ was 36 torr, and his base deficit was 21 mEq/liter. His arterial oxygen tension rose to 235 torr when he breathed 100% oxygen for 15 minutes. Intensive pulmonary care and other supportive therapy, as outlined in this chapter, were administered and the child regained consciousness six to eight hours following immersion (pHa 7.42, PaO_2 143 torr, $PaCO_2$ 38 torr, base excess = 0 at FIO_2 = 1.0). He continued to improve, except for persistent intrapulmonary shunting of blood through perfused but nonventilated alveoli, as was detected by arterial blood gas and alveolar-arterial oxygen gradient (A-aDO_2) determinations.[12] There was both persistent dullness to percussion and absence of breath sounds over the right lower chest.

An x-ray film of the chest, taken on the day following his near-drowning episode, showed the lower lobe of the right lung to be collapsed. Bronchoscopy was performed and solid food particles were removed from the right lower lobe bronchus. By a combination of hyperinflation therapy and chest physiotherapy, this area of the lung was subsequently reexpanded and the child made an uneventful recovery.

Progress made by a near-drowning patient, in regard to reestablishing normal ventilation-perfusion ratios and adequate oxygenation, should be followed by serial determinations of arterial blood gases and A-aDO$_2$. Even though the shunt through atelectatic alveoli may have subsided, it is frequently necessary to continue to provide the patient with an oxygen enriched atmosphere if hypoxemia is to be averted.[2,13] The duration of therapy necessary will vary considerably. Two examples follow: the first patient required oxygen therapy only briefly and, in retrospect, probably represents someone who *near-drowned without aspiration*. The second case is that of a woman who *near-drowned with aspiration* and required extensive pulmonary care for approximately six weeks.

Case 2

A five-year-old boy, when removed from the bottom of a fresh water swimming pool, was unconscious and motionless. He was treated with mouth-to-mouth ventilation and spontaneous ventilation began within one minute. En route to the hospital, he regained consciousness. During the admission interview, he was alert, oriented, and could recall jumping into the wrong end of the swimming pool (he could not swim). Arterial blood obtained while he was breathing room air showed pH 7.40, Pco$_2$ 32 torr, Po$_2$ 103 torr, and a base deficit of 5 mEq/1. A chest x-ray taken at this time was normal. His hemoglobin concentration was 12.8 gm% and hematocrit was 39 vol%. Serum electrolyte concentrations were: sodium 135 mEq/liter, chloride 101 mEq/liter, and potassium 4.2 mEq/liter.

The child was admitted to the hospital with a diagnosis of near-drowning without aspiration. Treatment consisted of supplemental oxygen using a face tent and intermittent positive pressure breathing therapy every four hours. The following morning, his arterial pH was 7.43, his PaO$_2$ was 91 torr, and his PaCO$_2$ was 27 torr (FiO$_2$ = .21). The low PaCO$_2$ probably reflected hyperventilation since the boy resisted and cried when stuck again with a needle. Treatment was discontinued and he was discharged from the hospital. He was still asymptomatic when followed in the out-patient clinic.

Case 3

A fifty-two-year-old white female accidentally drove her car into a fresh water canal. She was apneic when rescued and was given mouth-to-mouth resuscitation at the scene of the accident resulting in recovery of consciousness and spontaneous ventilation. On arrival to the emergency room, however, she was cyanotic, gasping, and unresponsive to verbal command. A physical examination showed a semicomatose patient who responded violently to painful stimulae; her blood pressure was 110/70, her pulse rate was 108/min., and her respiratory rate was 30/min. Her skin was mottled, had evidence of chronic dermatitis, and numerous abrasions were present. Her pupils were constricted, but equal and reacted to light. On auscultation, diminished breath sounds, rhonchi, and scattered wheezes were heard over the chest bilaterally. Later, it was learned that the patient had asthma, but that she had not required hospitalization for her disease.

Arterial blood was drawn on admission, while the patient was breathing oxygen by face mask; analyses showed: pHa 7.14, $PaCO_2$ 45 torr, PaO_2 68 torr. Venous blood was analyzed for concentration of serum chloride (88 mEq/liter), sodium (126 mEq/liter), potassium (3.9 mEq/liter), whole blood hemoglobin (15 gm%), hematocrit (45 vol%), and plasma hemoglobin (19 mg%). The patient was intubated with an orotracheal tube, and her ventilation was controlled with a ventilator which delivered 100% oxygen. Intra-arterial and central venous catheters were placed. Lactated Ringer's solution, steroids, isoproterenol, and antibiotics were administered intravenously. She was titrated with intravenous sodium bicarbonate against her base deficit (mEq bicarbonate $= 0.25 \times$ base deficit $\times$ kg), receiving a total of 360 mEq. She was admitted to the intensive therapy unit and, one and one-half hours after admission, her arterial blood pHa was 7.49, $PaCO_2$ 35 torr, and PaO_2 225 torr during controlled ventilation ($FiO_2 = 1.0$). Assisted ventilation was instituted two hours later, and the inspired oxygen concentration was adjusted to keep her arterial Po_2 between 70 and 120 torr.

Twenty hours after admission, her pHa was 7.55, $PaCO_2$ 32 torr, and PaO_2 122 torr with an FiO_2 of only 0.30. The following morning she pulled out her endotracheal tube. Arterial oxygen tension was measured after spontaneous breathing of 100% oxygen through a mask and nonrebreathing valve for 20 minutes; PaO_2 was 360 torr and $A-aDO_2$ was calculated to be 317 torr. The patient was maintained, thereafter, with oxygen via a nasal catheter and vigorous chest physiotherapy. Forty hours post aspiration pHa was 7.46,

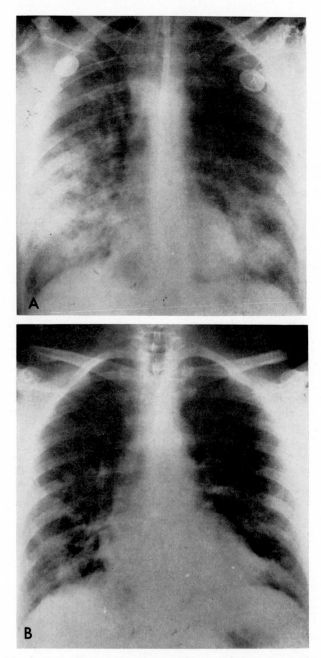

Figure 14. *A*, Xray film of the chest within one hour of near-drowning in fresh water. *B*, X-ray film of the chest sixty hours after near-drowning in fresh water shows considerable clearing from the admission film.

PaCO$_2$ was 37 torr, and PaO$_2$ was 175 torr. A culture of tracheal secretions taken on the evening of admission showed no growth. The x-ray film of the chest, taken 60 hours postaspiration, showed considerable clearing when compared to the film taken on admission (Fig. 14).

Eighty-four hours after admission, a marked increase in pulmonary infiltrate was seen on the chest x-ray (Fig. 15). Her rectal temper-

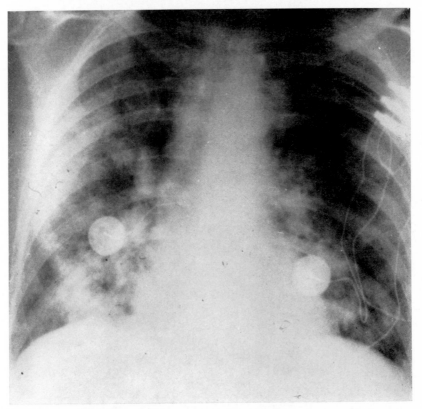

Figure 15. X-ray film of the chest eighty-four hours after near-drowning showing a marked increase in pulmonary infiltrate.

ature went up to 104.5°F, and blood gases drawn with the nasal oxygen catheter still in place showed severe hypoxia: PaO$_2$ 37 torr, PaCO$_2$ 27 torr, and pHa 7.53. She was given curare, was reintubated and ventilated mechanically with 100% oxygen at a tidal volume of 1,000 ml. After 20 minutes PaO$_2$ increased to 330 torr, PaCO$_2$ was 30 torr, and pHa 7.47. The patient was maintained with mechanical ventilation; the F$_I$O$_2$ ranged from 0.6 to 0.9 in order to maintain PaO$_2$ at approximately 80 to 120 torr. The pneumonia

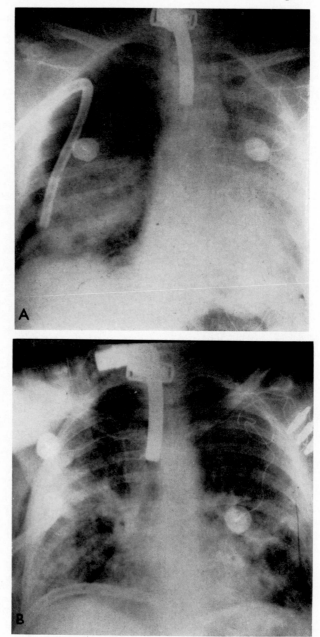

Figure 16. *A*, X-ray film of the chest showing recurrent tension pneumo-thorax of the right lung. *B*, The right lung is re-expanded after insertion of a second thoracotomy tube.

progressed. *Pseudomonas aeruginosa* was grown from her sputum on the eighth hospital day and antibiotics were adjusted according to sensitivity studies. A tracheostomy was performed over the cuffed nasotracheal tube. Two hours later the patient was in acute distress. A right pneumothorax was diagnosed and a thoracotomy tube inserted. The following day the chest tube stopped functioning suddenly and the patient turned deeply cyanotic. A recurrent tension pneumothorax was diagnosed and new thoracotomy tubes were inserted with immediate relief (Fig. 16).

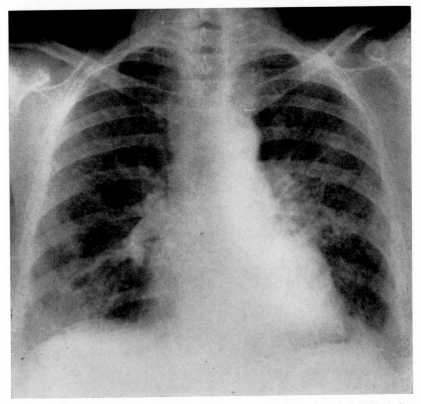

Figure 17. X-ray film of the chest taken on the thirty-eighth hospital day after treatment for near-drowning. This patient required mechanical ventilation for approximately five weeks.

Her course was "stormy" for the next few weeks. She was maintained with mechanical ventilation, alternating between assisted and controlled ventilation as the situation demanded. Inspired oxygen tension was varied according to that which was necessary to maintain a clear sensorium. It was noted that whenever her arterial oxygen tension dropped below approximately 60 torr, the patient became confused and disoriented, while above this level her sensorium was clear. For the most part, 50-60 percent oxygen was required to maintain this arterial oxygen tension. On the 26th hospital day, the patient could breathe spontaneously for short periods of time provided humidified oxygen (40 percent) was delivered via a "T" tube over the trachea; pHa was 7.38, $PaCO_2$ 47 torr, PaO_2 105 torr. Her tidal volume was 500 ml in a sitting position and vital capacity was 1,500 ml.

During the next ten days, she was weaned from the mechanical ventilator by gradually extending the period of spontaneous ventilation. Inspired oxygen tension was also gradually decreased until she could maintain normal arterial oxygenation on room air. Intensive chest physiotherapy and frequent use of a water aerosol produced by an ultrasonic nebulizer were necessary to assist in the removal of thick tenacious secretions. On the thirty-fourth hospital day, the tracheotomy tube was removed. Her lungs were clear, but breath sounds were slightly decreased throughout. She could cough up her secretions without difficulty. An x-ray film of the chest taken on the thirty-eighth hospital day (Fig. 17) showed only a slight increase in markings in the lower lobes and the patient was discharged from the hospital. Two months later, on a routine follow-up visit, her arterial oxygen tension was 79 torr while breathing room air and 467 torr while breathing 100% oxygen (pH 7.41, Pco_2 41 torr).

Occasionally, even in spite of intensive pulmonary care, the damage to the lung parenchyma is so severe that oxygen tensions necessary for survival cannot be maintained.[2,3] We could speculate that future hope for such patients may lie in long-term pulmonary bypass support. If the patient's blood can be artifically oxygenated for long periods of time, it is possible that these lung lesions may heal.

The above discussion on intensive pulmonary care assumes that the patient had an adequate circulation when admitted to the hospital. Obviously, if circulatory arrest is present, closed chest cardiac massage should be instituted along with pulmonary support and, in addition, an electrocardiogram must be obtained to determine whether or not the heart is arrested in asystole or ventricular fibrillation. If ventricular fibrillation is present, electrical defibrillation should be attempted immediately. A variety of drugs, including bicarbonate, epinephrine, calcium, and vasopressors have been advocated as adjuvants to external cardiac massage in an attempt to reestablish circulation.[14,15] Assuming that intensive pulmonary care has been started and circulation is intact, we are then in a position to complete the evaluation of the patient and provide total care.

MONITORING

Vital signs, e.g. pulse, respiration, blood pressure, and temperature, should be monitored in all patients who have suffered a near-drowning episode. If the patient did not aspirate fluid and regained consciousness soon after resuscitation was started, additional monitoring usually is unnecessary. If he aspirated fluid, however, his clinical status can change from moment to moment and extensive monitoring may be necessary. The electrocardiographic tracing and urinary output should be followed in all such patients. When difficulty is encountered in obtaining reliable arterial blood pressures by noninvasive methods, an intra-arterial catheter should be placed. The catheter can be threaded percutaneously into the radial artery in older children and adults. In turn, it is connected to a strain gauge and electronic recorder for continuous monitoring of intra-arterial blood pressure.

The arterial catheter also offers a reliable avenue for obtaining frequent blood samples for pH, Po_2, and Pco_2 determinations to guide treatment of ventilatory and acid-base status. While satisfactory arterial blood samples usually can be obtained by percutaneous puncture with a 25-gauge needle, an indwelling arterial catheter eliminates the possible hazard of basing treatment on blood gas and acid-base values inadvertently obtained on venous blood. This is of particular importance in patients where severe intrapulmonary shunting is present.

This author has treated a patient who had an arterial Po_2 of 27 torr while breathing 100% oxygen.[3] Since the sample was obtained percutaneously with a 25-gauge needle, the possibility of this having been venous blood was considered. An indwelling arterial catheter was placed and the reliability of the sample confirmed.

Overtreatment, based on mistaking venous for arterial blood, is also possible. An example of such a situation follows:

Case 4

A fifteen-year-old youth was playing with friends at the poolside when one of them put his arm around the youth's neck until he lost consciousness and threw him into a fresh water swimming pool. The patient was retrieved almost immediately, but was apneic on rescue. Mouth-to-mouth resuscitation was administered and he regained spontaneous ventilation and consciousness. He was awake when admitted to the emergency room approximately 30 minutes after his accident, but he answered questions very slowly. Vital signs were stable and respirations were unlabored at 12 to 14 per minute. Normal breath sounds were heard on auscultation of the chest, except for a slight decrease in intensity over the left lower lobe. A sample of heparinized blood was obtained by percutaneous puncture from what was thought to be the left radial artery: pH 7.34, Pco_2 40 torr, and Po_2 45 torr. Then he was given 100% oxygen to breathe. After 20 minutes of breathing 100% oxygen, repeat studies were performed by puncture of the same vessel and the Po_2 was reported as 60 torr. The A-aDO_2 of 613 torr, calculated from these values, indicated a severe absolute intrapulmonary shunt. This was not compatible with the clinical appearance of the patient. Therefore, a third attempt to obtain arterial blood was made by percutaneous puncture of the right radial artery. This showed an arterial Po_2 of 560 torr. Then, the patient was allowed to breathe room air and the sampling was repeated: pH 7.45, Pco_2 35 torr, and Po_2 84 torr. Further laboratory studies of hemoglobin, hematocrit, serum electrolyte, and plasma hemoglobin levels, and an x-ray film of the chest were all within normal limits. The patient was observed in the intensive therapy unit overnight and was encouraged to breathe deeply and cough frequently. Blood gas tensions of arterial blood, drawn the following morning, were within normal limits.

This patient probably was representative of a victim of *near-drowning without aspiration* or, at most, minimal aspiration, and required very little therapy. If treatment had been based on the initial blood gas values obtained, it is likely that the patient would have been intubated and his ventilation supported mechanically. In this case, the hazards of therapy based on the results of venous blood mistaken for arterial would likely be worse than the disease for which he was admitted. It is our practice that if the patient and the laboratory results do not appear to fit, and compatible results cannot be obtained within the first few moments of admission, a percutaneous arterial catheter is placed so that reliable guides for therapy can be obtained.

Data on blood volume changes in human near-drowning victims are not available, but these changes are likely similar to those of the animal studies summarized in Chapter V. It has been shown that it is difficult to quantitate the extent of blood volume change, particularly after sea water aspiration, because the commonly used tracers (serum albumin) may leak from the intravascular space, producing unreliable results. A more reliable method of assessing the physiologic response to circulating blood volume is to monitor the patient's central venous pressure (CVP). Catheters for monitoring CVP can be placed into the superior vena cava via percutaneous puncture of the external jugular vein, anticubital vein, or subclavian vein. We prefer to use the external jugular approach, since the tip of the catheter almost always can be placed in or near the right atrium and complications from this technique are minimal.[16]

The central venous pressure catheter also helps in evaluating the adequacy of myocardial function. Many near-drowning victims present with pulmonary edema, which is not secondary to circulatory overload but rather to a primary pulmonary injury. Under these circumstances, frothy edema fluid is present in the lung, but the central venous pressure is low. This is particularly true after sea water drowning when low central venous pressures reflect the hypovolemia caused by the loss of plasma into the lung. Rather than treating this type of pulmonary edema in the classic manner with fluid restriction, rotating tourniquets, morphine, and digitalis, these patients require fluid and volume replacement and an attack on their pulmonary edema via the pulmonary tree itself (e.g. intermittent positive pressure breathing and aerosols of antifoaming agents). Thus, the CVP helps differentiate between pulmonary edema from circulatory overload and that which is due to pulmonary injury. The availability of both CVP and arterial catheters also makes it possible to determine the cardiac output by the dye dilution method with little additional effort.

Rapid changes in body temperature can occur in patients after aspiration of fluid. It is helpful, therefore, to monitor temperature continuously with an indwelling rectal probe and read-out device.

Naturally, when the need to monitor a specific parameter is no longer present, the monitoring devices should be removed. This is particularly true of plastic indwelling venous and arterial catheters, since the hazard of infection and thrombophlebitis increases with the duration of time that they are left in place.

LABORATORY EVALUATION

The most important laboratory tests for an evaluation and guide to therapy of the near-drowning victim are the determinations of PaO_2, $PaCO_2$, pHa, and bicarbonate. Another related determination which is helpful is the alveolar-arterial oxygen gradient, measured while breathing 100% oxygen. This allows the physician to assess the degree of absolute or true intrapulmonary shunting.[2]

Even though severely abnormal serum electrolyte concentrations have not been reported in victims of near-drowning, electrolyte concentrations should be determined. If abnormal values should be found, specific therapy can be instituted. Whole blood hemoglobin and hematocrit and plasma hemoglobin levels also should be determined on admission to the hospital. They should be repeated at frequent intervals thereafter, until reasonable assurance of stability is seen. The whole blood hemoglobin and hematocrit values usually will be normal on admission to the hospital. After fresh water aspiration, however, there may be a decline in measured hemoglobin and hematocrit concentrations 12 to 24 hours after hospitalization. The reason for this has been discussed in Chapter VII. If the plasma hemoglobin level is not elevated on admission, it probably will remain normal throughout the hospitalization. If it is significantly elevated, steps should be taken to facilitate its elimination through a forced diuresis.

Although the arterial oxygen tension is a more reliable guide to therapy in the acute situation, roentgenographic examination of the chest may be helpful for comparison with follow-up films in the long-term treatment of these patients. The chest films will be helpful in determining the presence of complications such as the collapse of a lobe due to aspiration of solid particles, increasing infiltration due to infection, pneumothorax, or pulmonary edema. Also, it will demonstrate whether or not the patient's stomach was excessively distended, either by his swallowing water during the near-drowning episode or by the introduction of air during attempts at artificial ventilation by the rescuer. If gross gastric distention is seen on the film, steps should be taken to empty the stomach. This will usually improve ventilatory function.

DEFINITIVE HOSPITAL THERAPY

As stated earlier in this chapter, intensive pulmonary care must be continued as long as necessary in these patients. In some, it simply may be overnight observation and supplemental oxygen administration with deep breathing and coughing exercises. On the other extreme, patients have required mechanical ventilation for as long as five weeks after near-drowning. A detailed description of the methodology for prolonged mechanical ventilation is beyond the scope of this monograph. Suffice it to say that considerable attention must be paid to all aspects of mechanical ventilation, including airway maintenance, humidification, strict asepsis, adequate ventilation, judicious oxygen administration, appropriate selection of a ventilator, adequate assessment of ventilatory parameters, chest physiotherapy, care by a knowledgeable respiratory team, and rehabilitation. The reader is referred to other texts for details.[17,18]

If abnormal serum electrolyte concentrations are seen, specific correction by appropriate physiologic salt solutions is indicated. The most frequent abnormality seen in the clinical treatment of these patients is a low serum potassium concentration.[2] In general, intravenous fluid therapy should begin with the administration of lactated Ringer's solution and then be changed to the specific fluid required, based on the information obtained from laboratory results. Some authors have recommended the administration of hypertonic solution to all fresh water near-drowning victims and hypotonic solution to all sea water near-drowning victims.[19] Judging from the knowledge we now have about fluid and electrolyte changes in human near-drowning victims,[2] this type of routine therapy is without foundation and ill-advised.

If the central venous pressure is low, and other clinical signs indicate hypovolemia, administration of volume expanders and/or blood must be considered. After sea water near-drowning, blood rarely is necessary since there is not usually an extensive loss of red blood cells. On the other hand, volume expanders (e.g. Albumisol®) may be necessary to replace the plasma lost into the lung. After aspiration of large quantities of fresh water, hemolysis of red blood cells can occur. The extent of hemolysis may not be reflected in the whole blood hemoglobin and hematocrit concentrations on admission to the hospital. Serial determinations will sometimes show a gradual fall in these values. If sufficient red blood cells have been lost through hemolysis, the oxygen carrying capacity of the blood will be reduced and the patient may well derive benefit by replacement of whole blood.

DRUG THERAPY

The two most important drugs in the treatment of near-drowning victims are *oxygen* and *bicarbonate solution*. These two drugs should be administered routinely to all near-drowning victims. The necessity for continuation of such therapy should be based on serial determinations of arterial blood gases and acid-base balance. Broad spectrum antibiotics and parenteral steroids are indicated in all patients who have aspirated water.[10] If the patient's initial blood gas determinations are within normal limits, then it is doubtful that he has aspirated and antibiotics and steroids should be withheld. If proper attention is paid to balancing circulating blood volume with fluid replacement based on CVP measurements and urine output, vasopressor therapy rarely will have to be considered in these patients. Since vasopressors which stimulate the alpha receptors can further decrease tissue perfusion, the degree of metabolic acidosis seen in these patients can be compounded by their use. It may be advisable, on occasion, to employ drugs that work by stimulating the beta receptors to temporarily increase the cardiac output until blood volume can be stabilized. For similar reasons digitalis has been used to improve cardiac function during this very critical period. Prolonged use of any type of vasopressor agent is not indicated and, at best, these drugs are to be considered as a crutch rather than a specific mode of therapy.

Diuretics are helpful in promoting renal output, particularly in patients who have a high plasma hemoglobin concentration. While the agent of choice has been changing almost yearly, we are currently using either ethacrynic acid or furosemide when indicated.

Deliberately induced hypothermia also has been advocated in the care of near-drowning patients.[20] One rationale for its use is to decrease the oxygen requirements of the patient. In order to provide effective protection against hypoxia by decreasing the cerebral oxygen requirement, it is necessary to start hypothermia before the hypoxic insult. Obviously, this is not possible in the near-drowning patient. As a result, the rationale for the use of induced hypothermia can be questioned. On the other hand, if intrapulmonary shunting is so severe that arterial oxygen tensions necessary for adequate hemoglobin saturation cannot be maintained, then by reducing the oxygen requirement the small quantity of oxygen that is available can better supply the body as a whole. In this situation, it is imperative that pulmonary function and gas exchange eventually improve if the patient is to survive. Hypothermia also has been advocated as a method of decreasing cerebral edema. This may be helpful in patients who remain comatose in spite of the correction of arterial oxygen tension, pH, electrolyte and fluid balance.

Exchange transfusions have also been advocated in the therapy of fresh water drowning victims. An outstanding example of a patient treated this way is a child who was resuscitated after being submerged in frigid water for 22 minutes.[21] Unfortunately, laboratory results from blood drawn prior to exchange transfusions were not reported, so it is unknown whether his survival was the result of the exchange transfusions or in spite of them. Since approximately 85 percent of human drowning victims,[22] and presumably almost all near-drowning victims, aspirate 22 ml or less of water per kilogram body weight, severe hemolysis and electrolyte disturbance necessitating exchange transfusions rarely will be seen.

Summary

Near-drowning victims must be treated immediately for ventilatory insufficiency, hypoxia, and resulting acidosis. The success or failure of the overall resuscitative effort frequently will depend upon the adequacy of prompt intensive pulmonary care. These patients should have their fluid and electrolyte balance investigated and appropriate therapy started as indicated. Finally, the most important guide to the adequacy and type of therapy to be administered is serial determinations of arterial blood gas tensions, pH, and bicarbonate.

REFERENCES

1. Wong, F. M., and Grace, W. J.: Sudden death after near-drowning. *JAMA, 186*:724-726, 1963.
2. Modell, J. H.; Davis, J. H.; Giammona, S. T.; Moya, F., and Mann, J.

B.: Blood gas and electrolyte changes in human near-drowning victims. *JAMA, 203*:337-343, 1968.

3. Modell, J. H.: Ventilation/perfusion changes during mechanical ventilation. *Dis Chest, 55*:447-451, 1969.

4. Modell, J. H.; Gaub, M.; Moya, F.; Vestal, B., and Swarz, H.: Physiologic effects of near drowning with chlorinated fresh water, distilled water and isotonic saline. *Anesthesiology, 27*:33-41, 1966.

5. Modell, J. H.: The pathophysiology and treatment of drowning. *Acta Anaesth Scand Suppl, 29*:263-279, 1968.

6. Modell, J. H., and Moya, F.: Effects of volume of aspirated fluid during chlorinated fresh water drowning. *Anesthesiology, 27*:662-672, 1966.

7. Colebatch, H. J. H., and Halmagyi, D. F. J.: Lung mechanics and resuscitation after fluid aspiration.*J Appl Physiol, 16*:684-696, 1961.

8. Fuller, R. H.: The 1962 Wellcome prize essay. Drowning and the post-immersion syndrome. A clinicopathologic study. *Milit Med, 128*:22-36, 1963.

9. Modell, J. H.; Heinitsh, H., and Giammona, S. T.: The effects of wetting and antifoaming agents on pulmonary surfactant. *Anesthesiology, 30*:164-173, 1969.

10. Bannister, W. K., and Sattilaro, A. J.: Vomiting and aspiration during anesthesia. *Anesthesiology, 23*:251-264, 1962.

11. Hamelberg, W., and Bosomworth, P. B.: *Aspiration Pneumonitis.* Springfield, Thomas, 1968, p. 68.

12. Comroe, J. H., Jr.: *Physiology of Respiration; An Introductory Text.* Chicago, Year Bk Med, 1965, pp. 147-159.

13. Modell, J. H.; Moya, F.; Williams, H. D., and Weibley, T. C.: Changes in blood gases and A-aDO$_2$ during near-drowning. *Anesthesiology, 29*:456-465, 1968.

14. Jude, J. R., and Elam, J. O.: *Fundamentals of Cardiopulmonary Resuscitation.* Philadelphia, Davis, 1965.

15. Committee on Cardiopulmonary Resuscitation: *Cardiopulmonary Resuscitation. A Manual for Instructors.* American Heart Association, 1967.

16. Smith, B. E.; Modell, J. H.; Gaub, M. L., and Moya, F.: Complications of subclavian vein catheterization. *Arch Surg (Chicago), 90*:228-229, 1965.

17. Modell, J. H.: Basic principles of acute and chronic respirator therapy. In Banyai, A. L. and Gordon, B. L.: *Advances in Cardiopulmonary Diseases.* Chicago, Year Bk Med, 1969, Vol. IV, pp. 225-248.

18. Bendixen, H. H.; Egbert, L. D.; Hedley-Whyte, J.; Laver, M. B., and Pontoppidan, H.: *Respiratory Care.* Saint Louis, C. V. Mosby Co., 1965.

19. Shaw, C. C.: "Man Overboard." *Med Tech Bull, 7*:193-198, 1956.

20. Ohlsson, K., and Beckman, M.: Drowning—reflections based on two cases. *Acta Chir Scand, 128*:327-339, 1964.

21. Kvittingen, T. D., and Naess, A.: Recovery from drowning in fresh water. *Brit Med J, 5341*:1315-1317, 1963.
22. Modell, J. H., and Davis, J. H.: Electrolyte changes in human drowning victims. *Anesthesiology, 30*:414-420, 1969.

INDEX